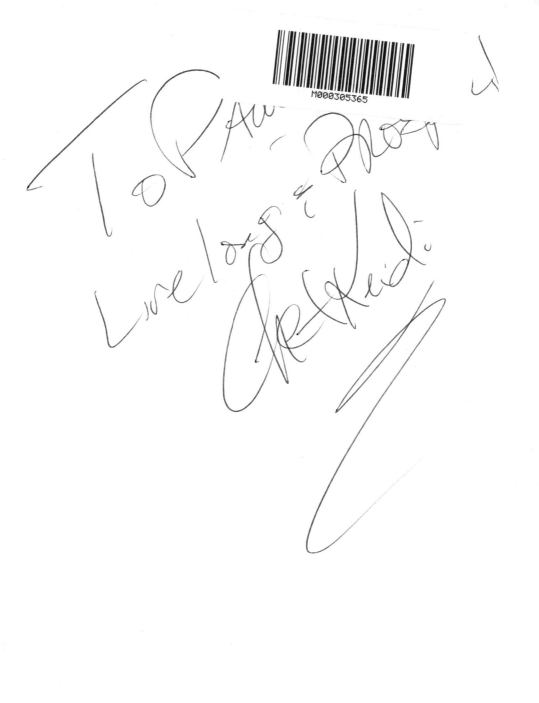

# LIVING SUPERFOOD LONGEVITY: Master the Possibilities of High-Quality Life Extension

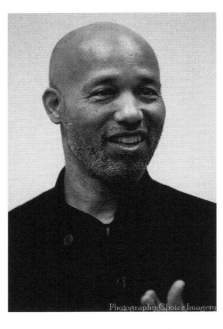

Photography Choice Imagery

This research report is authored by Keidi Awadu, aka The Conscious Rasta Copyright 2016 (Revised 2019) by Keidi Awadu

Published by the Conscious Rasta Press 9515 W. Cherrydale Ct., Las Vegas NV 89147 U.S.A.

The photo is courtesy of Choice Imagery, Baltimore

Library of Congress Cataloging-in-Publication Data is available from the publisher. This book, or parts thereof, may not be reproduced in any form without permission from the publisher; exceptions are made for brief excerpts used in published reviews.

This publication is designed to provide accurate and authoritative information regarding the subject matter covered. It is sold with the understanding that the publisher and author are not engaged in rendering legal, accounting, medical or other professional advice. If such advice is required, the services of a competent professional person should be sought whenever possible. Decisions made regarding the health of the reader are the sole responsibility of the reader and not the author and publisher of this book.

We have a wonderful set of DVD's to compliment this recipe book at www.LivingSuperFood.com. You can follow Chef Keidi at www.ChefKeidi.com. Be sure to sign up for our mailing list. Subscribe to my YouTube channel at https://www.youtube.com/c/keidiobiawadu

E-mail me (Keidi@chefkeidi.com) for those who want to book a workshop, catering session or Living Superfood demo, one-on-one nutrition consultation or other interaction on this wonderful new way of living and eating. The telephone number to reach my office is 323.902.2919 (10 AM to 6 PM Pacific Time)

## Table of Contents – LIVING SUPERFOOD LONGEVITY

# Introduction – Evolution and Devolution

Something truly historic and amazing is going on right before our eyes (actually, all of our senses) – Humanity is evolving. This transformation is taking place at an ever more rapid rate. We are getting taller, our brains larger, less susceptible to infectious diseases, living longer lives as well as being less-threatened by xenophobia (fear of others not like us) and forces of Nature. The pace at which this evolution is taking place has picked up dramatically over the slow pace of evolution that has affected homo sapiens over the past 3 million years.

Yet, this evolution is not happening consistently across the spectrum of humanity. For some, the outcome of this rapid transformation of our physical and mental well-being is going in a different direction. There are too many who are experiencing what might be considered *devolution* (de-evolution) with their brains atrophying due to excessive consumption of mass media (especially passive television viewing), their bodies suffering from excessive weight and obesity from the sedentary lifestyle, cardiovascular diseases, cancerous tumors, declining reproductive capacity along with a spectrum of immune and autoimmune disorders.

What is happening to the human species at this stage of our human existence is increasingly being determined by largely controllable environmental factors.

As I've become ever more obsessed with this subject of how, through deliberate lifestyle management, to achieve optimized, healthy longevity, I'll pose a question to people of how long they should want to, or expect to live. This dichotomy between what I call the *Evolutionaries* and the *Devolutionaries* is pretty telling regarding their response to this question. At this stage, within this society, a pessimistic outlook on life seems to have the statistical majority. When I talk about the rising number of centenarians (those now living to the age of 100 years and beyond) and inquire of people as to their thoughts on the subject, too often I get a negative response. Most of these responses have to do with the expectation that people of such advanced age are forecast to be dependent, handicapped, decrepit and miserable. As one accepts the all-too-frequently negative portrayal of the elderly within popular culture, becoming extremely old seems to be the most undesirable condition for most people. As well, nearly all of us have personal experience with dying grandparents or other relatives and don't want to imagine ourselves at such an advanced age as to undergo a similar end-of-life experience.

Then there are those conversations with what I am calling the "Evolutionaries" who are experiencing the more positive aspects of the progress of society and humanity. They see the possibilities of longevity as allowing more time to accomplish their life's mission, and for experiencing sustained vitality, health and prosperity in their lives. These tend to be the type of people who see all change as challenging, ripe with potential and opportunity. These people also tend to invest in short term behaviors which add to the likelihood of long-term gratification and a lifetime of reward.

I encounter Evolutionaries frequently among the extensive health consciousness communities within which I work and engage as a lecturer. Some people are very conscious of what they eat and drink, as well as minimizing the spectrum of environmental stressors to which they might become exposed. These people engage in healthy lifestyle activities including regular exercise, gardening, community involvement, and travel, along with a spectrum of creative and artistic endeavors. Thus, Evolutionaries easily envision having more years, decades even, of opportunity to enjoy the life that they are living.

Key to enjoying extra years of high-quality living is our ability to function without the burden of physical disorders and diseases. Sickness constricts our ability to engage with the world. Being *"sick and tired of being sick and tired"* does not enhance creative expression. Being *sick* is very expensive both in money spent on remediating symptoms of the disease as well as lost time due to constant distractions because of these disorders. Being *tired* limits one's ability to respond to, engage and challenge the spectrum of opportunities which Life offers.

Even worse, being sick and tired all the time is a major contributor to mental depression. From my own experience, depression is *antagonistic* to enjoying life to the fullest and the two mental states are nearly completely incompatible. As well, we do know that among the primary triggers for depression are malnutrition, poor health and lacking for vital energy.

This book is intended to take on this challenge of evolution versus devolution and to illuminate a *Golden Pathway* that each of us can commit to which will allow us to master all of the possibilities of *high-quality* longevity and life extension. The good news is that there is a lot of good news. A wealth of health science research is advancing across a spectrum of frontiers related to longevity. Within this study, we will look at many of these frontiers ranging from the obvious, such as nutrition, exercise, hygiene, and healthy relationships, to more obscure research that is rarely revealed within the media.

We will examine the world's longest living animal species, populations of long-living communities around the world, the complex interactivity among the body's metabolic systems, cellular biology, genetics, environmental stressors, and perhaps most importantly, the delicate balance between Mind, Body and Spirit which allows for longevity as well as quality in all of our relationships.

While many of us believe that optimal health, longevity and quality relationships should be a birthright afforded to all citizens of the world, this view is certainly not universal. The fact is that institutions ranging from governments, regulatory agencies, corporations, non-profits, media, and many healthcare institutions are uniting to present obstacles toward our being able to live healthy, thriving and creative lifestyles.

The profit motive among many competing businesses blocks the necessary sharing of the best ideas and information that could be used by the public toward an optimized lifestyle. There is little chance that this competition, greed, and abuse will disappear any time soon in the progress of society, thus it becomes necessary for those of us of a certain conscious awareness to forge our own pathways through this entangling morass of social, political and economic conflicts toward the aim of being self-determining toward all our enlightened self-interest.

It would be nice if we could rest assured that government regulatory agencies would stop these numerous assaults on our long-term health outcome. In an ideal world, corporations would base their profits on those things which have true benefit for their consumers. We can only imagine that the best information on disease remediation or prevention is what every scientist doing research in the field of healthcare has as the foundation for their careers.

Unfortunately, the contrary is all too common. Throughout my journalism career, I have documented these flagrant contradictions in a serious of books exposing *conspiracies and high crimes*. What has risen to dominate the economic and political functioning of the larger society often borders on blatant criminality. The oft-quoted social critic Christopher Hedges put these contradictions into perfect context with the following statement:

> "We now live in a nation where doctors destroy health, lawyers destroy justice, universities destroy knowledge, governments destroy freedom, the press destroys information, religion destroys morals, and our banks destroy the economy." [1]

This widespread trend of regulatory and institutional failure to protect the public is indeed a dilemma for the nation but it does *not* apply to everyone's circumstance. I am making the presumption that you, because of this book that you are currently reading, are a self-determining individual with a conscious awareness of how to pursue and achieve high quality, healthy living. Therefore, you and I have come to share this transformation. So, let's get this journey on its course. We have a very, very long and beautiful pathway before us.

The advice, information, research, and testimony that am sharing throughout this edition of the Conscious Rasta Report is intended for educational and inspirational purposes only. I am *not* a certified medical professional. I do *not* have millions of dollars in insurance to cover any errors that might occur should you follow my example and injure yourself. If you are suffering any manner of potentially life-threatening medical disorder, you should be in the care of a competent professional who is certified in his or her specific field of treatment.

I AM very good at what I do regarding natural health maintenance and disease prevention. These strategies have worked wonderfully for me for nearly 40 years since embarking on a plant-based dietary lifestyle. I

---

[1] Chris Hedges > Quotable Quotes, www.GoodReads.com

am very proud to tell people that, having surpassed my 60<sup>th</sup> birthday, I have *never* been on prescription drugs...NEVER! I have no medical issues other than very rare occasions of acute respiratory challenges (colds) and an occasional environmentally-triggered rash.

My own health tactics include the *7 Principles of Optimal Health*, which includes breath management, hydration, optimized nutrition, rest, exercise, detoxification and mind/spirit alignment. Since embarking on the extensive research that is included within this report I have accumulated a variety of nutritional supplements as well. For half of my adult life, I have also engaged in organic gardening. Another major component of my own foray into high-quality life extension is regularly expanding my mental power by studying and memorizing complex scientific research as well as learning new languages.

I consider myself to be very much an Evolutionary. As such, I strive to buck the trends that are popular or common within this society, such as indulgence in drugs, alcohol, pharmaceuticals, fast food, processed food and exposure to potentially toxic chemicals. I regard myself to be a living experiment in *conservation biology*. It has been a wonderful journey so far for the first half of my anticipated lifespan of 120 years. I hope you are inspired toward a long and vital life as well.

# Chapter 1 – Processes of Living Long and Healthy

## The New Centenarians

Many of us can vividly recall the unfortunate events that accompany the death of loved ones, parents, grandparents, siblings and even younger members of the family and community. Yet, most of us should also recall with exuberance the case of loved ones who lived to wonderful ripe ages. We speak glowingly of qualities that made them so remarkable in their senior years. We are quick to claim a likely genetic inheritance from those to whom we are related which will similarly allow us to enjoy robust and productive health during our own senior years.

How proud we are to claim that inheritance from someone who became a *centenarian* or lived well into their 90's as healthy, active, sharp of mind and graceful in their senior glory. These seniors inspire us with their healthy lives as well as their accumulated wisdom. For myself, and I am sure many of you agree, these Wise and Esteemed Elders are true *royalty* within our families. We celebrate them at family reunions and reserve prime space for them at family and community gatherings. We want to hug them with extra warmth, kiss their cheeks and assure them that they are treasured within our society.

Growing older with grace, wisdom, healthy and surrounded by loved ones is truly among the greatest blessings of a life well-lived. In our right mind, we would wish this upon all our parents, grandparents, siblings and community members. We should also wish this upon ourselves because we thus become a highly valued treasure for all of those who would benefit from you and me as their senior role models.

Longevity is truly a blessing and it is a blessing that we should lavishly wish upon ourselves just as we would lovingly wish it upon others.

Merriam-Webster dictionary defines *LONGEVITY* as 1) long duration of individual life, and 2) long continuance. Another online source, Dictionary.com adds further: 3) length of service, tenure, etc.; seniority. In the wellness community, we speak not only of extended years of life but emphasize the *quality* of those years, preferring to call this *healthy longevity*. The main aspects of healthy longevity include extended years of life, vitality, strong mental faculties, mobility and agility, independence from pharmaceutical medication, excitement for the golden years, ongoing accumulation of knowledge and wisdom, and continued reliable functioning of all of the body's systems.

The research that comprises this report mostly emerged from a month-long set of intensive studies that I compiled during my daily investigative research podcast on LIBRadio.com throughout the month of August 2015. This series was focused upon how each of us can dramatically extend our healthy, natural life expectancy, reduce the impact of chronic disease, have more energy, mental power and libido as we age gracefully.

The growing number of people living past age 100 affirms that steady progress in longevity research is being made, despite terrible pandemics of chronic disease that impact so many within the nation.

Thus, it serves each of us to comprehend the multiple factors that contribute to disease-proof living. From the "7 Principles of Optimal Health," to key nutrient classes, to the role of a spectrum of stressors in our lives, the ability to overcome environmental stressors and to enjoy a long and purposeful life is now within our conscious ability.

We do our best to contest the widespread perception that living long generally equates to prolonged suffering because the best data-based evidence suggests just the opposite. This is especially true for those who actively seek out and take on lifestyle habits that are conducive to high-quality life extension.

## Longevity Is Great Cause for Celebration

Born March 12, 1909, in South Carolina, Virginia McLaurin, a resident of Washington, D.C., had the chance to become a celebrated sensation on the event of her 107th birthday when she shared a meeting and videotaped dance at the Whitehouse with President Obama and the First Lady, Michelle. Arranged as part of Black History Month commemorations, the petite Mrs. McLaurin expressed such exuberance and joy for the moment that the president cautioned her to slow down. She explained the cause for her joy, "And I tell you, I am so happy. A black president. A black wife. And I'm here to celebrate black history. That's what I'm here for." Think about it... She lived these extra years for this moment.

The video went viral and the nation had a chance to share her joyous dance. So many times, when our most senior citizens perform such endearing feats of healthy longevity, it brings great joy to our hearts.

Another similarly impressive feat of longevity, former President George H.W. Bush celebrated his 90th birthday in 2014 by skydiving. President Bush, who had distinguished himself as a World War II fighter pilot, was no stranger to skydiving. Yet who among us would imagine or predict that such an elderly person, let alone a former president, would take on such a feat at such an advanced age. He shared the joy of his experience by sending the message, "It's a wonderful day in Maine – in fact, nice enough for a parachute jump."

Asian populations tend to produce significant numbers of *centenarians*, those living to age 100 and beyond. China's Bapan Village is also known as "Longevity Village." There a disproportionate number of centenarians have established the village as a medical phenomenon that has been examined by numerous teams of international researchers. While many researchers pursue the idea that the basis of such longevity is rooted in the genetic code, they do admit that likely no more than 25% of this longevity was due to genes, with the remaining 75% being a direct consequence of lifestyle. [2]

Residents of Longevity Village have distinct rural lifestyle characteristics that translate to longevity when matched to urban residents in China and other parts of the world. These include a high level of consumption of plant foods throughout the day, beginning with breakfast; physical activity well into their most senior years; as well as extensive social relations within multi-generational homes and throughout the village. The particulars of these lifestyle trends serve as the ongoing subject of research throughout this book and will be explored in much greater detail.

---

[2] 100 Years of Healthy Habits: Secrets of Chinese Centenarians, by Jennifer J. Brown, PhD, from www.EverydayHealth.com, April 2015

You are most likely reading this book for the purpose of learning more about these and many more secrets to optimal health and high-quality life extension. Longevity is a blessing that you not only get to enjoy for yourself but it is also shared by those loved ones around you. Your spouse, siblings, children, grandchildren, great-grandchildren, associates, community, township and nation all have the chance to celebrate your longevity along with you. Your wise elderly council also becomes a valued contribution to the larger society. For so many reasons, we can all be much better informed as we concern ourselves with making the best of our blessed years of life.

# Chapter 2 – **Longevity in Animals**

Toward the aim of understanding the complex life processes that contribute to longevity, scientists have engaged in innumerable studies of the biological processes that contribute to longevity. Some of these various species, inhabiting land, sea, and air, have such long lives that we should be quite impressed when we consider the numbers of year that they commonly accumulate.

Reporting for National Geographic, writing in her Weird & Wild blog in February 2014, author Jennifer S. Holland posted an article entitled *6 of the World's Longest-Lived Animals*, in which she named some of the oldest living species identified. [3] Among the six are the following oldest identified animals:

- A species of deep-sea clam that was named Ming, in reference to the Chinese dynasty during which it was born. At death in 2006, Ming was reported to have lived for 507 years and would have likely lived longer if it had not been accidentally killed by scientists "when they dredged it up off the coast of Iceland and froze it, along with many others, for transport back to the lab for climate change research." The blogger suggests that there are likely older living examples of the species known as an ocean quahog, *Arctica Islandica*, that have yet to be identified.

- A koi goldfish named Hanako died in 1977 and was believed to be 226 years of age. The species, whose age can be determined by counting its scales which are said to be linked to age like tree rings, normally living to be about 47 years old.

- Giant tortoises live in various parts of the world including the Galápagos Islands, mainland southern Asia, Australia, Indonesia, Madagascar as well as North and South America. The species is known for its longevity and there are several claims of specific tortoises whose life spans reached as high as 188 years (Tu'l Malila

---

[3] 6 of the World's Longest-Living Animals, by Jennifer S. Holland, Weird & Wild blog from National Geographic online, February 4, 2014

of Tonga Island), 150 to 250 years (Adwaita in India), and 176 years (Harriet, a Galápagos tortoise that died in 2006 at the Australia Zoo).

- Author Jennifer Holland also reports on "Immortal Jellies", a species of jellyfish, *Turritopsis dohrnii*, which was discovered in the Mediterranean region that "truly never dies," but recycles itself. The species is able to transmute "from an adult state to an immature polyp stage over and over again." Uncovering the secrets of this process may one day give humans a key to discovering a means of immortality.

There are other reports of long-living species. One report from *Forbes*, entitled "These are the Planet's Longest Living Animals," [4] lists the longest average lifespan among land and sea animals as:

1. Ocean Quahog (sea clam) – 400 years

2. Bowhead Whale – 211 years

3. Rougheye Rockfish – 205 years

4. Red Sea Urchin – 200 years

5. Galapagos Tortoise – 177 years

6. Shortraker Rockfish – 157 years

7. Lake Sturgeon – 152 years

8. Aldabra Giant Tortoise – 152

9. Orange Roughy – 149 years

10. Warty Oreo (fish) – 140 years

Around the world, many scientists are studying these and other species for cellular and biological processes which allow them to survive for so long. While these studies are appreciable toward unlocking many of the basic processes of life, we can derive certain facts from their existence that give us reason to adjust our lifestyle habits toward the same aim. With regard to land animals, there can be little doubt that the longest

---

[4] These Are The Planet's Longest-Living Animals [Infographic], by Niall McCarthy, Forbes Magazine, March 3, 2015

living species are plant eaters. Yes, it is true that, just like humans, plant-eating species live longer. These animals, which include tortoises, elephants, horses, and macaws all live primarily by consuming vegetables, grains, fruits and nuts.

A similar plant-focused diet is most closely associated with groups of long-lived humans within various cultures and nations around the earth. Later in this book, we will take an in-depth look at these various populations who enjoy longevity and embody certain lifestyle habits that best provide for high-quality life extension.

Ultimately, like these long-living animal species, environment and habitual patterns which facilitate a healthy lifestyle are keys to our optimal longevity. We will further discuss the many environmental conditions that might help or hinder our pursuit of long, productive, and active lifestyles. There are undoubtedly many differentials which impact our ability to resist diseases and accidents. Toward our pursuit of high-quality life extension, we will do our best to master as many as possible of the known lifespan-affecting variables.

As well, we aim to make this journey as enjoyable as possible.

# Chapter 3 – **Metabolic Syndrome and Longevity**

## How Compounded Diseases Impact Longevity

As a nutritional consultant, I am in regular discussion with people regarding intimate details of their personal health. Most often the discussion begins with one central disorder that has captured the client's attention for which an effective *natural* remedy is being sought. As I sketch a profile of that person's individual health status, what I am realizing more and more that, while there may be one particular area of focus, the problem entails multiple underlying conditions that have compounded, leading the client closer to the point of crisis.

A typical case might involve high blood sugar, *hyperglycemia*, which might have been labeled as diabetes or pre-diabetes. Yet, as the inquiry proceeds, I'm informed that this person is also on high blood pressure medicine (hypertension), for which the medicine is not alleviating the condition but merely suppressing symptoms. Common in such a case is also overweight or obesity (hyperadiposity), which itself can be commonly accompanied by clogged arteries (atherosclerosis), and abdominal obesity (visceral adiposity). What I am describing is, unfortunately, becoming more common among this generation which is suffering higher rates of non-communicable diseases (NCD's) than have previously impacted public health.

A compounding of such disorders is referred to as *metabolic syndrome* or sometimes referred to as "Syndrome X." The reliable online medical reference site WebMD has the following to share about the increasing rate of this diagnosis:

> Although it was only identified less than 20 years ago, metabolic syndrome is as widespread as pimples and the common cold. According to the American Heart Association, 47 million Americans have it. That's almost a staggering one out of every six people. The syndrome runs in families and is more common among African-Americans, Hispanics,

Asians, and Native Americans.  The risks of developing metabolic syndrome increases as you age. [5]

While metabolic syndrome is not necessarily considered a *disease* itself but actually represents a *disorder*, this collection of diseases is appearing more commonly within the increasingly troubling American public health status.

According to most health pronouncements, the diseases which comprise *metabolic syndrome* include the following:  high blood sugar, high blood pressure, excessive LDL cholesterol, a high triglyceride level, abdominal fat, and obesity.  As the syndrome's name implies, these are all conditions which are disorders of metabolism.  From my own perspective, this definition should also be expanded to other disorders which are part of metabolism, including progressive kidney disease (nephropathy) as well as an improper balance within the microbial flora of the intestinal tract; the *healthy* bacteria that are a critical component of our digestive process.

According to most diagnostic and treatment protocols, a person is diagnosed as having metabolic syndrome when they display symptoms of at least three of these conditions.

 While most of these 6 (or 8) diseases are largely relieved with appropriate lifestyle modifications when they begin to compound they lead inevitably to decreasing viability.  Throughout our studies, we will frequently repeat this central theme that we do not have to continue suffering from this particular set of compounding disorders.

Toward our further comprehension of the condition, for which specific preventative remedies will be shared, let us begin with the following from a broadsheet published by the U.S. National Institutes of Health / National Heart, Lung, and Blood Institute, entitled *What is Metabolic Syndrome?*

## Metabolic Risk Factors

Five of the conditions described below are most often listed as risk factors for diagnosis of metabolic disease.  My own research has

---

[5] What is Metabolic Syndrome?, from WebMD, www.WebMD.com

expanded this common listing of metabolic disorders to include progressive kidney disease as well as disruption of the gut bacterial balance. A person can suffer any of these indicators alone, but they tend to cluster together. If you have at least three of these disorders, you are considered to have *metabolic syndrome* also known as Syndrome X.

- **A bulging waistline** – This also is called abdominal obesity or "having an apple shape." Excess fat in the stomach area is a greater risk factor for heart disease than excess fat in other parts of the body, such as on the hips.

- **A high triglyceride level (or you're on medicine to treat high triglycerides)** – Triglycerides are a type of fat found in the blood.

- **A low HDL cholesterol level (or you're on medicine to treat low HDL cholesterol)** – HDL is most often referred to as "good" cholesterol. This is because it helps remove fatty plaque from your arteries. A low HDL cholesterol level raises your risk for cardiovascular disease.

- **High blood pressure (or you're on medicine to treat high blood pressure)** – Blood pressure is the force of blood pushing against the walls of your arteries as your heart pumps blood. If this pressure rises and stays high over time, it can damage your heart and lead to plaque buildup.

- **High fasting blood sugar (or you're on medicine to treat high blood sugar)** – Mildly high blood sugar may be an early sign of diabetes.

- **Nephropathy (kidney disease)** – This is a disease within the kidneys or damage to the kidneys caused by diabetes, adverse reactions to drug chemotherapies (i.e. AIDS nephropathy), toxicity or any manner of an inflammatory disorder.

- **Overweight/Obesity** – While it begs to argue whether excessive body mass index is causative or a symptom of metabolic disorders, there can be no denying that it often coincides with these diagnoses. *Hyperadiposity* can closely correlate with problems of digestion, cardiovascular disorders, and chronic inflammation.

- **Disruption of the Gut Microbiome (Clostridium difficile)** – We are seeing the rise of multiple digestive disorders which have their origin in the imbalance of the complex balance of an estimated 100 trillion mostly-friendly bacteria which inhabit our gut and aid in the digestion of food proteins.

We have born witness within recent decades to a dramatic rise in overweight and obesity within developed nations. This is accompanied by increasing diagnoses of metabolic syndrome. Rather than regard only one metabolic condition as a precursor or leading to others, from the perspective of a *holistic lifestyle*, we view them all as passengers on the same train. A diagnosis of metabolic syndrome is an indicator that the sufferer is in grave danger of decreasing quality of life and shortened lifespan. The presumption is that you are reading this book to avoid such a negative outlook for your life.

Throughout the book, we highlight strategies to avoid a diagnosis of these various conditions which comprise Syndrome X. The good news is, once again, that *there is good news*. Nearly all of these disorders have a strong correlation to lifestyle, nutrition, and exercise. Along with detoxification strategies, one can certainly secure one's own wellbeing.

The good news is that simple lifestyle changes can have a major impact as we commit to those habits that ensure health and longevity. Referring again to the link between diet and metabolic syndrome, we share this informative excerpt from the *British Journal of Nutrition*:

> The vegetarian dietary pattern is traditionally a plant-based diet that includes fruits, vegetables, cereals, legumes, nuts, vegetable oils, soya, and possibly dairy products and/or eggs. Vegetarians and other populations who follow a plant-based dietary pattern enjoy longevity. Specifically, vegetarian dietary patterns have been associated with a lower risk for developing IHD [Ischemic Heart Disease], type 2 diabetes, hypertension, specific cancers, lower all-cause mortality and reduction in cause-specific mortality. The prevalence of the metabolic syndrome (MetS) in the USA is approximately 20% and is currently increasing in developing countries in line with the obesity epidemic. The health care costs associated with the MetS are on a magnitude of 1·6 overall compared with healthy individuals, which makes it an important public health problem. Current evidence from several cross-sectional and case-control studies shows an association between

consumption of a vegetarian dietary pattern and a reduced prevalence or risk of developing the MetS. [6]

Note that from this excerpt that the authors imply that such a vegetarian dietary pattern might include "possibly dairy products and/or eggs." This is *not* consistent with vegan strategies for avoiding or overcoming the diseases associated with metabolic syndrome. We frequently state throughout the *Living Superfood* series that there are serious compromises *and* consequences in consuming these fringe *non-vegetarian* foodstuffs. Along with metabolic syndrome, a vegetarian or vegan diet is protective against a broad range of common diseases; the research we share herein supports such a determination convincingly.

I have one more important point about these conditions that comprise Syndrome X. As one engages procedures to alleviate one condition, other syndrome disorders begin to rapidly improve as well. As a nutritional consultant, I have worked with people whose intent is to overcome diabetes or excess weight with a typical 30 or 60-day strategy. They soon find that the first condition to reverse is generally high blood pressure. While we may be aware of relief of conditions which served as a foundation for disease, what is now occurring in the background is more complex. The body is now doing what it was designed to do and that is to repair, heal and normalize its own systems. This is accelerated by the diversion of regenerative energy away from fighting diseases and their symptoms toward restoring prime functionality through the body's multiple interrelated systems.

Ultimately, our studies advance toward the aim *and* process of affirming our ultimate goal of a rewarding longevity lifestyle. My hope is that we should all be excited with regard to this magnificent journey to wellness and a high-quality life extension.

---

[6] A Perspective on Vegetarian Dietary Patterns and Risk of Metabolic Syndrome, by Joan Sabate and Michelle Wien, from the British Journal of Nutrition, Vol. 113, April 2015

# Chapter 4 – **Oxidative Stress and the Aging Processes**

## Free Radicals, Inflammation, Antioxidants

Throughout this book, we will continue to revisit the central question as to what factors impact aging. Because the research and published literature on the aging processes are just so extensive, a comprehensive understanding of this central question is by necessity multifaceted. Some approaches are more along the lines of simple, natural living, while others require comprehensive insights into microbiological and biochemical processes. All along we will attempt to use practical anecdotes and lifestyle examples to illuminate this pathway toward high-quality life extension.

At this point, we look at a root cause of as many as 200 disease processes, including all of the major killers. They are all inescapably related to oxidative stress, which is itself a consequence of multiple factors including infection, malnutrition and environmental stresses. In this chapter, we will also share a spectrum of foods which are the best sources of *antioxidants* that go a long way to keep the body well balanced and highly functioning.

Back to the question of how and why we age. The journal *Oxidative Medicine and Cellular Longevity* describes itself as:

Oxidative Medicine and Cellular Longevity is a unique peer-reviewed, open access journal that publishes original research and reviews articles dealing with the cellular and molecular mechanisms of oxidative stress in the nervous system and related organ systems in relation to aging, immune function, vascular biology, metabolism, cellular survival and cellular longevity. Oxidative stress impacts almost all acute and chronic progressive disorders and on a cellular basis is intimately linked to aging, cardiovascular disease, cancer, immune function, metabolism and neurodegeneration. The journal fills a significant void in today's scientific literature and serves as an international forum for the scientific community worldwide to translate pioneering "bench to bedside" research into clinical strategies.[7]

I have long known that a significant portion of my audience is quite turned off by the peer-review scientific research process which supplies the foundation of what is an *evidence-based* scientific analysis. Yet, this very process has served as much of the core of what I contend should separate our comprehensive understanding of matters regarding science from the mass of hype, hyperbole, hysteria, unwarranted "spookism" and baseless conspiracy that has become all too pervasive in this era of Internet with its ubiquitous access to information from often-dubious sources.

During the course of studies which comprise this edition of the Living Superfood series, I came across the following peer-review study abstract which serves as a highly useful starting point for assessing the role of oxidative stress in our pursuit of high-quality life extension. Extracted from the pages of the journal *Oxidative Medicine and Cellular Longevity*, the following citation points out the complexities of achieving a comprehensive understanding of why we age:

### Redox Status and Aging Link in Neurodegenerative Diseases 2015 [8]

Aging is a multifactorial degenerative process and is characterized by progressive deterioration in physiological functions and metabolic processes, changes that drive numerous age-related disorders. Within cellular alterations are found oxidative stress, inflammation, and mitochondrial dysfunction, factors that converge in the aging and conduce to cognitive decline and other pathologies. Especially, the brain is susceptible to alterations in the redox environment due to its own properties (high concentrations of

---

[7] Oxidative Medicine and Cellular Longevity, About this Journal, Hindawi Publishing Corporation, New York

[8] Oxidative Medicine and Cellular Longevity, Volume 2015 (2015), Article ID 494316, http://dx.doi.org/10.1155/2015/494316

polyunsaturated fatty acids, high oxygen demand, and its poor antioxidant system compared with other organs). During the aging, the activity of antioxidant enzymes decreases and oxidative markers are elevated in various organs, particularly in the brain. This special issue contributes to an understanding of the mechanism involved during the aging process and provides the recent findings in this paradigm.

As I examine various points highlighted within this brief abstract of a much more comprehensive editorial, I realize just how difficult it is to convey the significance of the interactivity among such a broad spectrum of factors which are known to impact longevity. For the moment let us focus on comprehending this "Redox Status," the role of oxidation within the body's cellular processes, energy creation and what consequences can be expected when these processes get seriously out of harmony and order.

There are numerous terms which arise during this particular analysis that will require our understanding. For each definition we will attempt to make the descriptions as brief as possible:

- **Reactive Oxygen Species (ROS)** — This broad definition covers a number of biochemical processes involved in cellular energy formation and immune system function (generating the killing response to microbial invasion). ROS include a number of formations involving unpaired electrons, which result in unstable and highly reactive molecules, and also including superoxide, hydrogen peroxide, hydroxyl radical, nitric oxide and more. [9]

- **Oxidative Stress (OS)** — This is the resultant imbalance between the impact of the ROS system within the biological environment and residual toxic intermediates which must be cleared in order to prevent long term damage from reactive molecules to cell components, proteins, lipids, fatty acids, and DNA. Left unchecked, the presence of OS has been linked to a broad spectrum of age-related degenerative diseases, including cancer, Parkinson's disease,

---

[9] An Introduction to Reactive Oxygen Species - Measurement of ROS in Cells, 26-Jan-2014 / BioTek.com

Alzheimer's disease, diabetes, Sickle Cell disease, chronic infection, cardiovascular diseases, chronic fatigue syndrome and many other disorders associated with aging. [10]

- **Free Radicals** – This is the more common terminology used to refer to reactive oxygen species, the unstable oxygen molecules which control the undesirable microbial elements and pathogens impacting the body, as well as potentially damage vital cellular components. While free radicals are a critically necessary component of the body's immune system, unchecked they are major disruptors of the stable environment needed for long term health and stability throughout all the body's organs and systems. Free radicals can be an unwanted byproduct of bad diet, smoking, radiation, and other environmental stresses.

- **Antioxidants** – These comprise a spectrum of healthy chemical and nutritional compounds that are able to neutralize the impact of free radicals by capturing unbound electrons that make up reactive oxygen species. Antioxidants consist of vitamins, carotenoids, plant phenolics and other organic compounds such as ascorbic acid. Antioxidants are essentially pro-life and thus a highly desired nutritional component complimenting our optimized ideal of disease avoidance and the pursuit of longevity.

- **Redox Reactions** – The process by which the extra electrons represented by ROS are engaged during the oxidative process is referred to as redox, which "is a contraction of the name for chemical reduction-oxidation reaction." While these are fundamental chemical processes, they are ubiquitous throughout the spectrum of cellular life and thus constantly present within the normal function of biology. Ultimately the balance between redox reactions among free radicals and antioxidants gives us a strong determinant of the healthy normal functioning of immunity, detoxification, cellular protein functionality, DNA integrity and a spectrum of atomic-level functions within our microbiology. [11] Common redox reactions that we might readily recognize are corrosion and rusting, in which the oxidation of metal occurs in reaction to the presence of oxygen.

---

[10] Oxidative Stress, from Wikipedia, the free encyclopedia
[11] Redox, from Wikipedia, the free Encyclopedia.

- **Superoxide Dismutase-2 (SOD2)** – The SOD2 enzyme is just one of a number of important constituents of cellular signaling and the oxidative stress process. The metals iron and manganese, both key components of SOD2, are very important to the body's functioning, with both metals critical to the chemical structure of plasma and enzyme function, correspondingly. The role of these substances in energy production within the cell is extremely important and quite complex. Superoxide dismutase (SOD) is an example of the spectrum of enzymes which are catalytic agents that trigger a vast spectrum of life processes that are dependent upon sub-cellular chemical activity. Specifically, the SOD2 enzyme is critical towards programmed cellular death, oxidative stress, the life-cycle of the cell's mitochondria and normal tissue cell homeostasis. [12]

- **Mitochondrial Function** – So very much of our quest toward health, life processes, cellular integrity, and longevity involves energy production within each cell. The chief energy-generating component is called the mitochondria, the "little engine that can" which exists within each cell. This fuel generator works in a manner quite similar to other internal combustion engines across technology, basically utilizing oxygen and fuel (glucose) to create energy in the form of adenosine triphosphate (ATP), which then drives virtually all internal biological processes which are energy-dependent. Because the process is so overarchingly related to the spectrum of oxygen-dependent processes, it is definitely in our best interest to comprehend and to optimize these mitochondrial functioning processes toward the goals of long life, disease resistance, and maximum energy production efficiency.

- **Inflammation** – In preparing notes for these brief explanations of critical components of our cellular systems which are central to oxygen utilization and energy creation, the special significance of inflammation cannot be over-appreciated. Yet, connecting the relationship of inflammation to aging could itself become topic of a very extensive volume – a book unto itself. Inflammation's role in aging encompasses a number of sub-topics including the central question of "cause, effect, or both?", redox stress, mitochondrial

---

[12] Cell Death: Critical Control Points. By Danial & Korsmeyer, from Cell Journal, Vol 116, Issue 2, Jan. 2004

functionality, immunosenescence (immune system aging) as well as endocrinosenescence (endocrine system aging), and a cascade of other critical metabolic functions. [13] As this larger publication continues to unfold, we will examine as many of these different aspects of the inflammation-aging connection as can be compressed into this particular volume. To say the least, a comprehensive understanding and optimized management of the many inflammatory processes presents as the greatest area of active management wherein our efforts will be rewarded with high-quality life extension.

- **Antioxidant Foods** – Later in the book we will have much more to share on the topic of "Superfoods to Charge the Immune System"; a diet that is loaded with natural food antioxidants. The list here will thus be kept short, as it needs to be, because the optimal antioxidant-rich diet is as simple as eating a broad array of fresh fruits and vegetables in the least-processed state as is possible, especially organic and raw. Top performers in this category include dark grapes, blueberries, goji berries, dark chocolate (without excess refined sugar and milk proteins), pecans, artichokes, kidney beans (must be soaked, drained and cooked to avoid *antinutrient* tannins), cranberries, blackberries, cilantro, and various citrus fruits.

From this point on, our studies will become more focused on narrow areas which are related to our intelligent pursuit of longevity. All along, primary emphasis will be on those factors which are not only powerful environmental modulators of life processes, but are also key areas where specific tactics, techniques, and habitual changes allow you and I greater advantage in securing our goal of longevity and enhanced physical performance.

We have been born in a most opportune generation, one in which a spectrum of science, technology, knowledge accumulation and natural elements all can complement the rapid acquisition of high-quality life expectancy.

---

[13] Inflammation in Aging: Cause, Effect, or Both?, by Nancy S. Jenny, Discovery Medicine Journal, June 2012

We strive to be representative of a generation of wisdom, resourcefulness, creative focus and excitement about these frontiers of human capability. As such, we enthusiastically bring forward as many of our talents, resources, and opportunities toward the expression of the Greatest Good that can be imagined and developed for the benefit of ours and future generations.

High-quality life extension is so much about *quality living* itself. This includes quality of relationships, application of our collective resourcefulness, the valuing of self-sacrifice while at the same time being living examples of an overall *joie de vivre* (joy of living). The actualization of that which contributes to this joy is what I hope you gain as the main takeaway of this book. As well, I want to show by living example, that which I present to you herein is one of Life's greatest and rewarding engagements: high-quality life extension.

# Chapter 5 – **Reviewing: *The Blue Zones*, by Dan Buettner**

Most of my followers are aware of my years of ongoing daily Internet radio broadcasts on www.LIBRadio.com. As well, for most of this long history, we have set aside Monday's broadcast for intensive book study sessions. One of the many books which have excited our audience was **THE BLUE ZONES: Lessons for Living Longer from the People Who've Lived the Longest**, by Dan Buettner.

While we did engage in extensive study of Dan Buettner's book during our study series on the webcast, for the purpose of this analysis we will summarize as briefly as possible our studies to highlight a few of Buettner's most impactful lessons on longevity, as well as leading more fulfilling and disease-free lives. These insights include more than the obvious points on nutrition, diet, and exercise. For many people, it is *seemingly* peripheral lessons regarding spiritual expression, community belonging, personal goal-setting and other matters of the heart that will serve as keys to transformative lifestyle habits that induce longevity and quality of life.

Buettner's book began as a 2005 cover story article for *National Geographic Magazine*, entitled "Secrets of Living Longer," which qualified as a finalist for that year's National Magazine Award. Examining four particular populations around the world known for longevity and disease avoidance in more advanced senior-aged populations, "The Blue Zones" refers to longevity-associated population clusters in Okinawa Japan, Sardinia Italy, Costa Rica, and Loma Linda California. This research highlights a collection of lifestyle patterns common to these regions whose people have become associated with high-quality life extension. The book features numerous inspiring examples of individual lives and personal habits of memorable characters with which the author has spent significant personal time.

My work as an author is largely depending on the *meta-analysis* of research from others whose efforts are institutionally supported and thus able to be more comprehensive and nuanced. I most certainly appreciate these detailed personal profiles that Buettner and his colleagues have assembled. Yet, because of my own extensive experience of hands-on engagement with a spectrum of biological sciences over the decades, I am able to share additional insights and points of analytical focus that I trust you can appreciate. Sometimes it is our comprehensive understanding of the best work of other researchers that allows us to appreciate our own capacity for understanding. We each can contribute to the great body of knowledge that comprises a generation's collective contribution to the advance of wisdom within society.

Nine central themes that Buettner's research in *The Blue Zones* center upon include: 1) natural movement (exercise) in daily activities; 2) caloric restriction ("Hara Hachi Bu" in Japanese); 3) a dietary core centered around plant-based foods; 4) moderation in alcohol consumption; 5) a purpose-driven life; 6) stress-reducing habitual patterns; 7) spiritual faith expressed daily; 8) extended family support; and 9) membership and an active participation within the "right tribe."

As stated before, we so often focus narrowly on diet, exercise, and stress when we consider issues of longevity. Here I want to focus more on *The Blue Zones'* research into spiritual expression, community, personal goal setting and other matters of the heart as they all relate to high-quality life extension.

As the author stated in introducing his book and this research:

> A long, healthy life is no accident. The secrets to longevity are widely debated and sometimes misunderstood – yet remarkable groups of people manage to achieve it naturally, enjoying longer life spans while remaining active and vital well into their 80s, 90s and 100s. These people can be found in the world's "Blue Zones," extraordinarily long-lived communities where common elements of lifestyle, diet and outlook have led to an amazing quantity and quality of life. [14]

---

[14] The Blue Zones: Lessons for Living Longer from the People Who've Lived the Longest, by Dan Buettner, from the back cover text.

Here are choice excerpts from Buettner's book which correlate to four lifestyle patterns which have become associated with longevity and quality of life during one's senior years.

### LESSON FIVE: PURPOSE NOW

> Okinawans call it *ikigai* and Nicoyans call it *plan de vida*, but in both cultures, the phrase essentially translates to "why I wake up in the morning." The strong sense of purpose possessed by older Okinawans may act as a buffer against stress and help reduce their chances of suffering from Alzheimer's disease, arthritis, and stroke. [15]

For most of us this idea of living with purpose sounds simple yet practical; the French call it *raison d'être*. Still, as we are directing our focus on how lifestyle contributes to measurable longevity, it serves to expand our further awareness of these concepts. A strong purpose in life marshals resources deep within the soul, the conscious and the unconscious mind. The human experience is richly resourceful and, because of the phenomena called *the placebo effect*, we know that within the body is the ability to defy physical logic and to produce outcomes which could be regarded as miraculous.

Some key points that Dan Buettner points out on this topic of purposeful living during our senior years include:

- "It was also reported that immediately following December 31. 1999, demographers saw a spike in deaths among elders. These older people, in other words, may have willed themselves to stay alive into the new millennium."

- "A sense of purpose may come from something as simple as seeing that children or grandchildren grow up well. Purpose can come from a job or a hobby, especially if you can immerse yourself completely in it."

---

[15] The Blue Zones, Pg 245

- "A New activity can give you purpose as well. Learning a musical instrument or a new language gives you a double bonus, since both have been shown to help keep your brain sharp longer."

- "Craft a personal mission statement. If you don't have a sense of purpose, how do you find it? Articulating your personal mission statement can be a good start."

- "Find a partner. Find someone to whom you can communicate your life purpose, along with a plan for realizing it."

Thus, living with purpose, a vital plan for life and enthusiasm for specific future goals are definitely among the many facets of life for which we seek mastery. It is widely reported that for a significant portion of the older population, the course of health deterioration and death accelerates upon retirement. To the contrary, those who are highly motivated, see themselves as vital to the interests of the larger community, and have strong motivation toward future accomplishments, manage to hold onto their vitality and they remain enthusiastic for opportunities to fulfill their most important future achievements. The best part about this "plan de vida" is that it is directly within our control; it is a motivating factor which each of us can claim for our own advantage.

### LESSON SEVEN: BELONG

Healthy centenarians everywhere have faith. The Sardinians and Nicoyans are mostly Catholic. Okinawans have a blended religion that stresses ancestor worship. Loma Linda centenarians are Seventh-day Adventists. All belong to strong religious communities. The simple act of worship is one of those subtly powerful habits that seems to improve your chances of having more good years. It doesn't matter if you are Muslim, Christian, Jewish, Buddhist, or Hindu. [16]

The author points out that elderly people who regularly attend religious services, even if only once a month, can reduce their risk of death by about a third. He points out a study of Seventh Day Adventists, funded

---

[16] Ibid, Pg 251

by the National Institutes of Health, which followed some 34,000 people for 12 years, and "found that those who went to church services frequently were 20 percent less likely to die at any age." Linking this spiritual devotion to chronic diseases, Buettner concludes: "It appears that people who pay attention to their spiritual side have lower rates of cardiovascular disease, depression, stress, and suicide, and their immune systems seem to work better." [17]

He points out that a number of lifestyle traits, healthy behaviors, and personal disciplines tend to accompany those who are regular practitioners of spiritual faith. "They were physically more active, less likely to smoke, do drugs, or drink and drive. People who attend church have a forced schedule of self-reflection, decompression, and stress-relieving meditation..."

The author suggests several strategies we can take away from this valuable lesson of faith and belonging:

- "Be more involved. If you already belong to a religious community, take a more active role in the organization."

- "Explore a new tradition. If you don't have a particular religious faith, commit to trying a new faith community. If you don't' subscribe to any specific denomination, or if you haven't found a positive religious experience, you may want to explore a belief that is not based on strict dogma."

- "Just go. Schedule an hour a week for the next eight weeks to attend religious services... Studies show that people who get involved with the service (singing hymns, participating in prayers or liturgy, volunteering) may find their well-being enhanced."

There can be no debate that faith and belonging enhance life throughout an entire lifespan. Making this an important strategy later in life, toward the aim of increasing high-quality life expectancy, offers a valuable tactic each us can adopt. We are essentially spiritual beings in the first place. Therefore, incorporating spiritual expression into your community life makes good sense on so many levels.

---

[17] Ibid, Pg 252

**LESSON EIGHT: LOVED ONES FIRST**

*Make family a priority*—The most successful centenarians we met in the Blue Zones put their families first. They tended to marry, have children, and build their lives around that core. Their lives were imbued with familial duty, ritual, and a certain emphasis on togetherness. This finding was especially true in Sardinia, where residents still possess a zeal for family. I asked the owner of one Sardinian vineyard who was caring for his infirmed mother if it wouldn't be easier to put her in a home. He wagged his finger at me, "I wouldn't even think of such a thing. It would dishonor my family." [18]

*The Blue Zones* has much to say on the topic of putting family priorities first. Buettner points out a number of facts that confirm the critical importance of family love and support, each of which we can see a great advantage to the elder members of the family. As well, much of this devotion is also extended to family members who have already transcended into death and become ancestors. Common among those inhabiting Blue Zones around the world is the rejection of putting elderly family members into group homes or assisted-living facilities. As the Sardinian agriculturalist put it: "It would dishonor my family."

Among critical lessons from this section of the book:

- "All 99 inhabitants of one village were descended from the same 85-year-old man. They still meet for meals at a family-owned mountaintop restaurant, and the patriarch's grandchildren still visit him daily to help him tidy up or just to play a game of checkers."

- "Okinawans over 70 still begin the day by honoring their ancestors' memories. Gravesites are often furnished with picnic tables so that family members can celebrate Sunday meals with deceased relatives."

- "Their children check up on their parents, and in three of the four Blue Zones, the younger generation welcomes the older generation into their homes. Studies have shown that elders who live with their children are less susceptible to disease, eat healthier diets, have lower

---

[18] Ibid, Pgs 254-255

levels of stress, and have a much lower incidence of serious accidents... America is trending in the opposite direction. In many busy families with working parents and active kids, family time can become rare as everyone's schedules become more and more packed with things to do. Shared meals and activities can drop off the daily routine, making time together difficult to come by."

Buettner closes this section with four essential strategies, which are in brief: 1) Get closer; 2) Establish rituals; 3) Create a family shrine; and 4) Put family first.

These are undoubtedly all very good suggestions. Growing up in America, most of us have seen this discontinuance of family centeredness that has taken place in the last half-century. Numerous rituals which traditionally contributed toward family solidarity have become less commonplace and the number of households which no longer have reserved space for elders has skyrocketed; this is not civilized. It is thus no wonder that people in old-age homes and assisted-living facilities die lonely, depressed, medicated and neglected. We can certainly do better than this.

### LESSON NINE: RIGHT TRIBE

This is perhaps the most powerful thing you can do to change your lifestyle for the better. For residents of the Blue Zones it comes naturally. Seventh-day Adventists make a point of associating with one another (a practice reinforced by their religious practices and observation of the Sabbath on Saturdays). Sardinians have been isolated geographically in the Nuoro highlands for 2,000 years. As a result, members of these longevity cultures work and socialize with one another, and this reinforces the prescribed behaviors of their cultures. It's much easier to adopt good habits when everyone around you is already practicing them. [19]

We earlier examined the longevity benefits of belonging and religious affiliation. Humans, like many other species, are by nature social beings. Many studies on sociology, anthropology, and the biological sciences

---

[19] Ibid, Pgs 257-258

point out this correlation between social connectedness and high-quality life extension. The author cites a Harvard University study that "found that those with the most social connectedness lived longer. Higher social connectedness led to greater longevity" and that people "with the least social connectedness were between two and three times more likely to die during the nine-year period of the study..."

Further, when looking at chronic disease conditions that negatively impact our quality and length of life, this correspondence to social connections remained prominent. Citing an article from the *New England Journal of Medicine*, Buettner points to a study of over 12 thousand people who were tracked for 32 years wherein it was noted that "subjects were more likely to become obese when their friends became obese. In the case of close mutual friends, if one became obese, the odds of the other becoming obese nearly tripled. It seemed the same effect occurred with weight loss." [20]

As well, it must be noted that women are more likely to be beneficiary of social support networks, which likely accounts for a significant contribution toward women's average lifespan advantage over men. Citing Dr. Robert Butler, "They have better and stronger systems of support than men, they're much more engaged with and helpful to each other, more willing and able to express feelings, including grief and anger, and other aspects of intimacy."

Buettner closes with the following tactics for creating a supportive social network:

- Identify your inner circle – "Know the people who reinforce the right habits, people who understand or live by the Blue Zone secrets."

- Be likable – "Of the centenarians interviewed, there wasn't a grump in the bunch... Likable old people are more likely to have a social network, frequent visitors, and de facto caregivers. They seem to experience less stress and live purposeful lives."

- Create time together – "Spend at least 30 minutes a day with members of your inner circle. Establish a regular time to meet or share a meal together."

---

[20] Ibid, Pgs. 258-259

Throughout this excellent book *The Blue Zones: Lessons for Living Longer from the People Who've Lived the Longest*, the author Dan Buettner has much, much more to contribute to our treasure of knowledge toward gaining an advantage during the process of maturity.

One of the great takeaways from the book is that we can push aside the notion that growing old need be a period of suffering, chronic debilitation, depression or lack of enthusiasm for the days, weeks, months and years that will come to pass. To the contrary, as one reads this book, one is filled with hope as the lives of these centenarians are shared in detail. These longevity-blessed individuals, families, and communities are enriched in so many ways by these beloved Elders.

You and I must consider our intrinsic value to our children, grandchildren, great-grandchildren, extended family, community and nation as we grow older, wiser, more compassionate and beloved within the social network. Throughout this book, I seek to point out not only the tactics, science, and practices which equate to longevity, but as well highlight the true value of becoming cherished elders within our sphere of love and influence.

We want to be as valuable as possible to our family, community and to the world at large. We don't want to grow into a burden without commensurate reward. We want to contribute to the proper governance and shepherding of the society toward its greatest potential.

I hope that you, after having read this chapter, will be motivated to acquire a copy of Dan Buettner's book for your family's library – and read it as well. This is the type of book that would make a great gift to family members, friends and associates as well; certainly, you want as many as possible within your circle of compassion to share your healthy longevity with you.

The practical knowledge packed within this bestselling book will only contribute positive value to your life successes and family integrity. I can assure you that my vision for longevity will motivate me to frequently revisit *The Blue Zones* for inspiring tactics.

# Chapter 6 – **Supercharging Your Immune System for the Future**

## The 7 Principles of Optimal Health Revisited

Now that you've built up a bit of momentum with these studies, we can turn up the level of scientific engagement and stretch the boundaries of our comprehension just a bit more. In other words, the learning curve will get just a little steeper as we continue with this research. Key concepts for this chapter's focus include: natural immunity; the critical role of oxygen in the evolution of the human biology; more on reactive oxygen species and redox processes; full-spectrum nutrition; bio-systems compatibility; epigenetics; and the application of knowledge-based systems for sustainability.

We find ourselves in a most promising yet unquestionably *contradictory* moment in history. Today's accumulated wisdom stems from the most ancient of civilizations and is a legacy for which all of us should be inspired and tremendously grateful. The origin of ancient Egyptians' scientific wisdom can be traced to the *prehistoric* birth of Nile Valley civilizations. Bridging that legacy up to today's frontier of data-driven science, we can now bear witness to a vast accumulation of knowledge that should sustain health, societal progress, and sustainable prosperity. This progression of wisdom should also sustain optimism about the future which lies ahead.

Yet the split between those humans who are evolving while others are devolving is a paradox to which we must apply our scientific insights.

Compared to the earliest forms of simple bacterial life (*prokaryotic*), one-half billion years of the progressive evolution of life on Earth has led Homo sapiens (thinking man) to become incredible complexes of oxygen-dependent cells (*eukaryotic*). This places humanity at the apex of a 500-million-year long chain of evolutionary achievement. Our bodies represent an amalgamation of 50 trillion cells which are energetically compelled to cooperate toward the creation of an optimized vehicle for our soul's occupation within a cycle of life lasting for *as long as 120 years or more* at this stage of our evolution.

Yet the other part of this paradox is awareness of the tremendous burden that "modern society" has placed upon our species. Too many of us, as individuals, families, and communities, are currently shouldering a disproportionate burden of disorder, disease, self-limiting psychology, as well as a widespread sense of anxiety regarding our fate.

At our best, we are self-determining, resourceful, proud, confident and cognizant of our abilities to manage whatever challenges lie ahead. As such we strive to be mindful of the spectrum of empowering toolsets which have been developed for the benefit of ours and future generations. Each individual, a dynamic expression of the ongoing evolution of all species, should be present in the world as the greatest of a long line of genetic greats. Ours is truly a generation standing upon the shoulders of giants as we reach ever closer to the stars.

Correspondingly, the highly-evolved human immune system is a product of 500 million years of cell differentiation, genetic refinement, adaptive evolution, and thus has the *potential* to represent the most responsive and capable resistance against diseases that has ever arisen among all species on the planet. The potential for high-quality life extension is now increasing at the fastest rate documented in the modern scientific era. In the past two centuries, whole societies have witnessed much of the elimination of premature death due to infectious diseases such as rheumatoid fevers, pulmonary infections, water-borne parasitic diseases, childhood infections, and unmanageable inflammatory processes.

Yet, in contradiction to this positive momentum of our understanding of Nature is the appearance of a whole new spectrum of man-made immunological threats. These can range from antibiotic-resistant bacterial infections to industrially-produced-food-borne superbugs, reports of suddenly-appearing vicious pandemics of Ebola, HIV/AIDS, Zika virus, or the periodic announcement of some ethnically-evolved or cross-species pathogen (i.e., *Asian flu, avian flu*). For many of us within natural health scholarship, media-fed hysteria over these exotic bugs is generally hyped way out of context with respect to the *actual dangers* which are posed by the overuse of antibiotics, chemicals in the food chain, toxic exposures from pesticides as well as grave dangers from a spectrum of environmental stressors, ranging from personal care products to industrial chemicals.

Amidst these and other threats, real or imagined, you and I are tasked with the mission of making the absolute best of the spectrum of increased capacities which accompany our critical mission in this time of human progress. Quite simply, we've got to be as smart as our collective intelligence can manifest, and as resourceful as would be the result of our inheritance of the accumulated wisdom of humanity.

Ongoing studies show us that a plant-centered nutritional lifestyle (that of an *herbivore*) has proven itself superior to that of the *ultra-omnivorian* society within which we have been reared. An average American omnivore will eat essentially anything marketed as "food" by the nation's profit-obsessed corporations. People eat whatever is on television, despite the fact that our biological systems have not evolved compatibility with this gross, overly-processed dietary conflagration.

So many Americans take their primary cues as to what constitutes acceptable nutrition from commercial advertisements throughout mass media. It seldom matters to such people that the fundamental laws of nutrition for humans would follow the same universal rules of nutrition for other species. With other primarily vegetarian animals, such as elephants, rhinos, hippopotamuses, and gorillas (all of whom are large, plant-eating mammals), the thought that they could remain healthy while eating like humans might seem an obvious absurdity. Yet, within modern societies, logic is often convoluted with regard to maintaining the integrity of human nutrition.

Is there anyone among us who could think that a captive gorilla whose diet would become dependent upon excessive calories from junk food, burgers and fries, sodas, sweets, highly processed and chemical-laden food, would remain strong, live long and resist disease? We might never consider such for the gorilla, a vegetarian mammal, yet too often we unconsciously subject our children to such a terrible nutritional fate.

For humans to enjoy optimal health through nutrition, our diet must be constructed upon a foundation of consuming foods which facilitate oxygen-dependent metabolic processes, supply proper hydration, and supply an abundant spectrum of critically important nutrients. These critical nutrients consist of: protein, carbohydrates, amino acids, essential fatty acids, fiber, minerals, vitamins, and enzyme-rich unprocessed food. When the integrity of these critical nutrients is achieved through a wholistic diet, then the effective functioning of all of our body's synergistic systems can be better achieved.

As much as any of the body's systems, the *immune system* is the primary beneficiary of our wise and disciplined behavior. As such, contrary to habits which feed epidemics of inflammatory diseases within the larger society, we can create the right environment whereby the burdens of infectious disease, inflammation, metabolic disorders (i.e., diabetes, overweight, abdominal obesity, hypertension, etc.), as well as energy imbalances can all be avoided due to our conscious application of self-empowering habits and techniques.

We will need *supercharged* immune systems to fend off assaults from superbugs that are expected to continue to emerge from this larger corrupted environment. Today, within the U.S., some 24,000 people die each year from *antibiotic-resistant bacteria* that are mostly the byproduct of a combination of the nation's food supply system (especially meat from Concentrated Animal Feeding Operations, so-called *CAFO's*) as well as increasing danger from staph infections from the nation's hospitals and outpatient centers, where antibiotic overuse is feeding this crisis.

The humans naturally evolved a complex system for overcoming infectious pathogens which science refers to as *reactive oxygen species (ROS)*. This encompasses an expanse of processes, including oxidative stress, free radicals, and antioxidants, which occur within what we call *redox reactions*. Detailing the complexity of this endogenous (created within the body) system for ridding the body of dangerous pathogens would itself demand a significant amount of explanation for one's complete understanding.

We can state that this ROS system has intelligently evolved over the course of hundreds of millions of years for complex, oxygen-dependent cellular life on Earth. The contradictory idea that man's recent technical advance of synthetic biochemistry pushing into mimicking these basic life principles might supersede a half-billion years of biological selection, is *not* supported by the best available evidence. To the contrary, the appearance of a growing number of notoriously-dangerous antibiotic-resistant superbugs in recent decades stands as the best testament that synthetic biochemistry is *not* an optimal strategy for disease avoidance. Modern antibiotics will continue to have their place but should be limited as much as possible to infrequent short-term response to life-threatening bacterial challenges.

To gain our best advantage within this gradual process of human evolution, we can integrate as much as possible a spectrum of naturally-selected processes for our integration into a natural biological order. The following **7 Principles of Optimal Health** can serve as good guidance toward the goal of supercharging our natural immune systems in order to avoid so-called *superbugs* of the future.

- We are the product of 500 million years of oxygen-dependent cellular evolution. Mastering a spectrum of breath management techniques will bring great advantage to immune system functionality, stress-management, and epigenetic direction over our biological systems;

- The existence of life on this planet is directly related to the presence of water and its fundamental correspondence to life. Optimized hydration is thus absolutely critical to the maintenance of all health processes. Maintaining the highest integrity of the water we consume is paramount to healthy longevity;

- Optimized nutrition requires constant access to the spectrum of critical nutrients in their most digestible forms possible. This not only requires that we access, vitamins, minerals, the full spectrum of amino acids, essential fatty acids, fiber, complex carbohydrates, proteins, and enzyme-laden raw foods, but that proper preparation of our food demands that we do not harm the integrity of these nutrients through improper preparation techniques;

- Our immune systems are rejuvenated through periodic rest and, as such, we mustn't deprive our body of its daily requirement for proper sleep;

- Exercise is fundamental toward balance within a whole-body oxygen-dependent matrix as well as for ensuring that circulatory, muscular and skeletal systems are functioning optimally. All processes that constitute enhanced immunity are reinforced with the right types of regular exercise: cardiovascular, strength training, as well as stretching and balance exercises;

- An accumulation of a spectrum of toxic stressors always accompanies the rise of inflammatory processes within the body. Therefore, toxin avoidance, detoxification and the efficiency of waste elimination are all keys to strong immune functioning;

- Our best comprehension of complex, yet subtle, interaction within the Mind-Body-Spirit matrix requires that we pay particularly close attention to both psychological and spiritual processes that would serve our wholeness. While the commonly held understanding that "you are what you eat" has great merit, still, we are much more than what we eat and drink. We are how we think, interact, conceptualize, actualize, laugh, cry, empathize and create within the larger circle of Earth species. We are faith-bound Spirits within a multiplicity of material worlds and as such, must consider that our active and co-creative engagement with Nature is key toward manifesting our greatest health potential.

Yes, we all deserve by mere birthright, health, prosperity and high-quality longevity yet these will not necessarily manifest by default. These outcomes demand conscious awareness, investment of creative energy, study, practice, mastery, and ongoing reinforcement. As we master the progress of evolution and cumulative accomplishment, then it makes sense that each of us strive to be the *best human* that has ever been born.

Ultimately, we can best give proper grace and respect to the notion of a "Great and Mighty Creator" by *being* the *body of creation* through constant real-time activity in this world throughout our lives. How fantastic might it be to have an amazing discovery, at that final moment of our corporal existence, that we were, in fact, our own Great and Mighty Creator all along?

# Chapter 7 – **Why We Age; A Review of Gary Null's Power Aging**

*"What causes aging? The easy answer to that question is the uncontrollable passage of time. But aging is also the result of a number of biological and pathological processes that vary from person to person and are controllable to some degree, with existing therapies... So understanding the biological processes involved can really pay off..."*
— Dr. Gary Null, PhD [21]

Among my favorites of the numerous books which we have examined during our Monday book study broadcasts on LIBRadio is **GARY NULL'S POWER AGING: The Revolutionary Program to Control the Symptoms of Aging Naturally**. Dr. Gary Null, PhD had authored more than fifty books by the time of publication of *Power Aging*, and is considered by myself and many others as the premier researcher in the nation on matters of natural living, drug-free means of overcoming chronic disease, critiquing peer-review scientific journal health research, as well as presenting critical insights into the value of vitamins and nutrition supplements for our strategy to stay disease free.

If one searches for Dr. Gary Null's research on the Internet, you will notice that he is frequently condemned by adherents to the mainstream medical authority of the American Medical Association (AMA). Why would establishment-supporting critics engage such a castigating attitude toward naturopathic practices as developed by one of the best health researchers of the generation? Because, quite simply, Null's conclusions nearly always go contrary to notions of widespread vaccinations, drug therapy, the cancer orthodoxy, and the efficacy of many of the most common practices of the largely-for-profit medical

---

[21] GARY NULL'S POWER AGING: The Revolutionary Program to Control the Symptoms of Aging Naturally, Pg 43

industries. I am in 100% accord with the stance that Gary Null has taken on these and other matters and consider him to be perhaps the strongest influence on my own evolution toward science-based, data-driven and evidence-based knowledge on health issues.

Hence for me, this book *Power Aging* stands as a treasured compilation of cutting-edge research. Within this book, Dr. Null takes a near-360-degree exploration of every topic that could be possibly related to longevity, with special attention toward the numerous ways that our behaviors, habits, and practices can impact our ultimate longevity outcome. This book is about allowing you control over your destiny.

In Chapter 3 of Null's book, entitled "**WHY DO WE AGE? The Biological Processes of Aging**," the author cites *The Life Extension Foundation* as a source of much of the information on the mechanisms of aging that is covered in this extensive chapter. I am as well a longtime subscriber to the monthly journal published by this health sciences research group. Much of the following, excerpted from this chapter, are based on both Null's and the Life Extension Foundation's research into the mechanisms of aging.

- **WHAT TELOMERES TELL US** – "…DNA will facilitate only about sixty to eighty cell replications, with variations depending upon the particular organ involved. As they approach the end of their programmed life spans, older cells divide less rapidly and less efficiently. Today scientists are furthering our understanding of this process of cell senescence by taking note of the structures called telomeres; these are small fragments, composed of DNA, that form the protective ends of chromosomes. What scientists are seeing is that with each new cell division, the telomeres are shortened, and that after these structures shrink down to a certain size, cell division stops. In other words, telomeres are a kind of biological clock, with decreasing length indicating a decreasing amount of cell lifetime left. ¶ "But what if we could replenish shrinking telomeres? …A naturally occurring enzyme called telomerase has been discovered and what it seems able to do is copy the telomeres' RNA in the form of DNA, and then put it on the ends of chromosomes, thereby extending cell life." [22]

---

[22] Ibid, Pt 44

- **FREE RADICALS** – "If your skin is aging prematurely and you are suffering from cataracts—both common conditions associated with advancing years—the culprit could be the free radical... ¶ "After a free radical is formed, it seeks to rebalance itself by taking an electron away from another molecule. Sometimes it can accomplish this within a harmless chemical reaction. But sometimes, in its quest to get an electron from another molecule, the free radical will inflict molecular damage. Thus normal enzymes, proteins, and cells are destroyed... When DNA is attacked by free radicals, for instance, genetic mutations result, and are passed down, a situation that can result in cancer." [23]

- **OXIDATIVE STRESS** – "It is important to note that free radical formation accompanies normal and essential biological processes and, thus, can never be fully eliminated... But while we cannot eradicate the free radical, we can control it. This is where antioxidant foods and supplements come into play. Antioxidants can latch on to free radicals and neutralize them. Unfortunately, few people eat enough antioxidant foods or take the proper combination of antioxidant supplements to adequately compensate for age-induced loss of endogenous antioxidants... Furthermore, most of us in this society eat foods that speed up the production of free radicals, such as saturated fats. Plus in the process of consuming more calories than we need, we are producing more free radicals than we need to." [24]

- **HORMONE IMBALANCES** – "The trillions of cells in the human body are delicately synchronized in their functioning by chemical modulators called hormones. Hormonal imbalances are often a contributing cause of many conditions associated with aging, ranging from new patterns of fat distribution, loss of libido, and increased fatigue to depression, osteoporosis, and coronary artery disease." [25] Gary Null goes on to point out further the critical importance of a spectrum of hormones which decrease as our bodies age, necessitating supplementation toward replenishing hormone levels we benefited from in younger years. These include DHEA

---

[23] Ibid, Pg 45
[24] Ibid, Pg 46
[25] Ibid, Pg 48

(Dehydroepiandrosterone), insulin, testosterone and a group of estrogen hormones.

- **CHRONIC INFLAMMATION** – "Another factor that you could call both causative of aging and associated with it is chronic inflammation. We all know that aging people suffer an epidemic of outward inflammatory diseases, such as arthritis. But chronic inflammation also does interior damage—to brain cells, arterial walls, heart valves, and other structures in the body. Heart attack, stroke, heart valve failure, and Alzheimer's disease have been linked to the chronic inflammatory cascade that so often afflicts aging people." [26]

Within this section of the association between chronic inflammation and age-related disorders and disease, Dr. Null goes on to further point out links to a spectrum of inflammation markers and specific disorders. Among the various biological processes which reflect this connection, he goes deeper into inflammation markers such as fibrinogen, C-reactive protein, pro-inflammatory cytokines, and homocysteine. Throughout this book, we will have more to say about these specific inflammation-associated blood markers.

Other keys to answering the critical questions of why we age are highlighted in Gary Null's chapter on the topic, for each of which he does provide detailed information. These other mechanisms include: DNA mutations, immune system dysfunction, glycosylation ("...a devastating chemical reaction... wherein protein molecules bind to glucose molecules in the body to form nonfunctioning structures") [which is analogous to the process of forming advanced glycation end products (EDC's) and carcinogenic substances called *acrylamides*], methylation deficit [methyl is necessary for proper DNA expression], mitochondrial energy depletion, excessive calcification, fatty acid imbalance, digestive enzyme deficit, excitotoxicity, circulatory deficit and our age-associated thoughts and attitudes.

To say the least, this chapter is highly informative and *GARY NULL'S POWER AGING* should present itself to you as inspiring, informing and authoritative as you increase your practical knowledge of the aging process and how to interrupt age-related physical degeneration. If I can

---

[26] Ibid, Pgs 46-47

use my own expansion of health awareness, cutting edge natural science, and comprehension of the great deficiency of western medicine, this book should serve you equally as well as a powerful tool within your longevity arsenal.

# Chapter 8 – **Why We Age; Review of Andrew Weil's HEALTHY AGING**

In this chapter review, we share insights from noted health scientist Dr. Andrew Weil, M.D. taken from his book **HEALTHY AGING: A Lifelong Guide to Your Physical and Spiritual Well-Being**. Key insights from this book allow comprehension of longevity factors such as "carmalization" of food substances within our bodies that results in the formation of dangerous *Advanced Glycation End Products (AGE's)* and other heat-generated byproducts that accompany unnatural eating styles. Other key takeaways from Dr. Weil's book instruct us about the role of sugar and other refined carbohydrates, cross-linked proteins (lipofuscin) and other damaging agents that are nearly all largely avoidable as we focus on health and refine our lifestyle habits.

Dr. Weil begins this chapter with the following paragraph:

> There are many theories as to why we age. Some focus on the accumulation of errors in the genetic code, others invoke loss of telomeres. You don't need to know the details of all of these theories, but I thought it might be interesting to review two of them to give you a sense of the ways researchers are thinking. The first has to do with a chemical process called caramelization, and the second concerns oxidative stress. Both have practical import, the former because it suggests that dietary changes may reduce the risk of age-related diseases, the latter because it raises questions about whether we should take antioxidant vitamins and minerals in order to preserve youthful health and function as long as possible. Both theories suggest that senescence and longevity are separable, that age-related disease is not a necessary consequence of aging. [27]

---

[27] HEALTHY AGING: A Lifelong Guide to Your Physical and Spiritual Well-Being, by Andrew Weil, M.D., from the chapter Why We Age, Pg 66

Dr. Weil explains this process of *caramelization* by drawing a comparison to the same process used in the culinary arts of combining "mixtures of sugar, cream, corn syrup, and butter to make caramel candy" and other such caramelization effects used by chefs. While the browning of foods, the creation of crusts, and other caramelized food effects are considered desirable by food connoisseurs, when it comes to optimized nutrition and natural eating lifestyle concerns, caramelization effects represent significantly dangerous processes. When sugars and proteins are combined at higher cooking temperatures, beginning from about 250 degrees Fahrenheit, they form chemical bonds which are called *advanced glycation end products (AGEs)* or alternatively referred to as *acrylamides (acrylic amides)*, which are proven to be quite harmful to our health.

The author cites the groundbreaking research of Dr. Anthony Cerami, "a medical researcher and inventor and member of the National Academy of Sciences," and his advancement of a "glycation theory of aging." Weil writes:

> It postulates that reactions between proteins and sugars in the body eventually form a class of compounds called "advanced glycation end products." Or AGEs for short. AGEs can damage other proteins as well as DNA and RNA. They do so by fostering abnormal bonds between adjacent protein strands, a change called "cross-linking." Cross-linked proteins are deformed—less elastic, less flexible, and less able to perform their normal functions." [28]

We cannot overlook the critical importance of what is being revealed here. Many of the favorite foods within the Standard American Diet (S.A.D.) are based upon combining proteins and sugars at increasingly higher temperatures. These include bread, toast, French fries, mac & cheese, pastries, fried and baked foods, barbecue and many, many more commonly eaten foods. Weil continues this warning within the same paragraph:

---

[28] Ibid, Pt 69

...It is cross-linking that makes the proteins in the lens of the
eye turn opaque to form a cataract.  Cross-linked proteins
account for the wrinkling and sagging of old skin.  Cross-
linked proteins in blood vessels are the basis of
arteriosclerosis, hardening of the arteries.  Cross-linked
proteins in the brain may contribute to the development of
neurogenerative diseases like ALS, Parkinson's, and
Alzheimer's.

He goes on to point out numerous other ways that AGEs and cross-linked
proteins put our health in danger as they are associated with causation
of a spectrum of diseases and disorders.  Among the many perils that Dr.
Weil points out are included increased risk of inflammatory and
autoimmune responses, increased cell proliferation (the basis of cancer),
hypertension, kidney disease, retinopathy, osteoarthritis, and most
assuredly "all the complications of diabetes."  A plethora of health
dangers has been identified that can be traced to the high amount of
AGEs in the S.A.D. diet.

Dr. Weil explains further regarding the dangers with the denatured food
that has become common within the modern diet, to which can be
attributed to many stress-inducing effects:

In addition to creating an overabundance of food in modern
society, we have also changed the nature of many foods,
refining and processing them from their natural state into
forms that interact with our systems in new ways.  This is
most problematical with carbohydrate foods.  Instead of
eating our grains in whole form—parched, boiled, or chopped
and cooked into chewy, chunky porridges—we mill them into
flour, discarding the fibrous hull and oil-rich germ.  This
pulverized starch is digested very rapidly, causing spikes in
blood sugar and corresponding surges in insulin secretion
that, over time, lead to loss of sensitivity to that hormone in
those with thrifty genes...  And, of course, our diets are now
flooded with sugar itself, something the pancreases of our
distant ancestors never had to deal with.  They got sugar only
in ripe fruit and an occasional honeycomb.  We get it in almost
every meal, especially in foods and drinks flavored with cheap

sweeteners made from corn. This dietary change favors glycation and the formation of AGEs. [29]

All throughout this book I will have much to say regarding the corruption of the modern diet and associated increased risk of developing chronic disorders such as hyperglycemia, diabetes, metabolic syndrome and the proliferation of inflammation, all stemming from high levels of consumption of refined carbohydrates. Of them all, refined sugar is unquestionably among the top offenders, with bleached flour following closely.

As this critical analysis of the factors that promote aging continues, the author shares the following alarm about *age spots*, which he regards as markers for the advance of cellular damage:

> You know those "age spots" that most people develop and that doctors tell us have no significance? Actually, they may have a great deal of significance, because the same material that composes them gets deposited in many places that are not visible, including the brain. The name of this brown age pigment is *lipofuscin*, derived from the Greek root for "fat" and the Latin root for "dusky" or "dark." The term is inaccurate, at least the "fat" part. Lipofuscin is not one substance but a heterogeneous mixture of fats, proteins, and metals, especially iron. It is waste material, the consolidated debris of worn-out cellular structures that cannot be eliminated easily from the body, and it piles up inside cells, particularly ones that are no longer actively dividing. That includes heart muscle cells and nerve cells.
>
> Clearly, lipofuscin is a marker of age. It starts to accumulate right after birth and continues to do so throughout life at an accelerating rate. We still don't know whether it is a cause of aging or a result of it, or whether cells stuffed full of it suffer damage from it... ¶ Other experts think that lipofuscin is a product of the interaction of cellular waste with free radicals, the highly reactive molecules generated by damaging

---

[29] Ibid, Pgs 70-71

oxidation reactions. It is also possible that when large amounts of age pigment are packed into cells, the cells become more susceptible to oxidative stress. [30]

This bridges our analysis of *Healthy Aging* into the second major take away from this chapter on "Why We age," and that regards Dr. Weil's insights into the impact of *oxidative stress*. As we did cover this topic extensively in Chapter 4, we will share just a few of the author's own views of the critical role of this redox process and the advance of aging.

After explaining many of the same basics relative to *reactive oxygen species (ROS)* that we have already covered, Dr. Weil compares the impact of "free-radical chain reactions" to radiation exposure, stating:

> "In fact, this is exactly the mechanism of radiation poisoning. Exposure to radiation, whether from X-rays or nuclear explosions, breaks down water in our bodies, generating free radicals that damage DNA, proteins, cell membranes, and other vital structures. The symptoms of radiation poisoning— immediate gastrointestinal havoc, later loss of hair, and, much later, development of bone cancer and leukemia—are consequences of that free-radical damage. [31]

Certainly, all of us in our right minds should be greatly concerned about exposure to radiation and its impact on both short term and long term health. The similarity between radiation damage to a similar impact from oxidative stress and free radical damage should be equally disturbing. Very few of us go through our days, weeks, months or years with the subject of oxidative stress occupying our active consciousness. Yet, from the perspective of pursuing a high-quality life extension, we should undoubtedly allow more focus on the impact of oxidative stress and related subjects.

Dr. Weil further explains the absolute impact that constant exposure to OS has on our health:

---

[30] Ibid, Pgs 72-73
[31] Ibid, Pgs 74-75

Oxidative stress is simply the total burden placed on organisms by the constant production of free radicals in the normal course of metabolism, added to whatever other pressures come from the environment. The latter include natural and artificial radiation; toxins in the air, food, and water; and miscellaneous sources of oxidizing activity, such as tobacco smoke, one of the most concentrated delivery systems of free radicals.[32]

He continues, citing the important connection between oxidative stress and longevity:

A good case can be made that health depends on a balance between oxidative stress and antioxidant defenses. Senescence [programmed cellular aging] and the appearance of age-related diseases represent the inability of antioxidant defenses to cope with oxidative stress over time with the steady accumulation of defects in DNA, in proteins, and in membranes. From this point of view, "senescence" and "longevity" are not synonymous. IF antioxidant defenses are strong, long life without disease should be possible. Certainly, this is the case with some centenarians, who enjoy good health until near the end, then decline rapidly. Most people would like to age that way, and if more of us could do it, we might not have to worry so much about the economic consequences of greater longevity. If the oldest old were to remain relatively disease free, their impact on the health-care system might not be so great, even if there were many more of them in a population. [33]

Before we close our analysis of this insightful chapter from a highly-respected natural health expert, let's share just a very brief instruction toward practical actions that one can take to offset the damaging risks from excessive oxidative stress.

---

[32] Ibid, Pg 76
[33] Ibid, Pgs 76-77

> Go into any health-food store, drugstore, or supermarket, and you will find a great many antioxidant supplements for sale, including vitamins C and E, beta-carotene, green tea extracts, resveratrol, curcumin (from turmeric), and Pycnogenol (from the bark of a pine tree)... [34]

I further offer the option of Living Superfood as Nature's *most perfect medicine*, which is the dominating theme of my own philosophy toward healthy aging.  Throughout the spectrum of plant-based foods, antioxidant nutrients can be acquired in great abundance.  We will have much more to share about the details of full-spectrum hyper-nutrition as an ideal longevity solution in later chapters.

I do highly recommend this book *Healthy Aging* by Dr. Andrew Weil.  It has served up an enlightening education for me and I trust that you will also find it insightful and inspiring.

---

[34] Ibid, Pg 78

# Chapter 9 – **Caloric Restriction, S.A.D. Food, and Aging**

In this chapter, we look at the body of data showing how *eating less* is associated with disease resistance and longevity. The primary mechanism here is an advantageous shift in the redox system, a part of natural immunity which, if imbalanced, creates damaging free radicals.

Here we have an abundance of good news from the frontier of longevity research. Among clinical and observational studies that are producing positive results is the theme of *caloric restriction (CR)*. As Dr. Andrew Weil put it, "...in warm-blooded species the only proven method of life extension is restriction of caloric intake, an intervention sometimes called 'caloric restriction with adequate nutrition.'" [35]

As we will clearly detail in this chapter and throughout this book, we can take advantage of caloric restriction as a longevity tool yet the value of "adequate nutrition" cannot be compromised. Toward this end, an optimized nutritional lifestyle, combined with systemic detoxification and other beneficial habits of healthy living, must all be coordinated to our highest capability. When we get the right balance of the eight critical classes of nutrients within a diet that is minimized for toxic stresses and receive these nutrients in the least-degraded form possible (i.e. raw, vegan, organic, fresh and enzyme-laden), then we can obviously eat less and still obtain the best nutrition. This optimization is key to our longevity success. Herein we will share reliable research to prove it true that by eating better and eating less, we can live longer.

My own experience investigating the impact of caloric restriction includes a significant number of analyses of peer-reviewed science. These publications consistently reveal the close association of caloric restriction (CR) with a lower risk of cellular, protein and DNA damage from oxidative stress. Correspondingly, there is a definite association between higher levels of food consumption and the proliferation of damaging free radicals. This collection of study literature also shows that

---

[35] Healthy Aging, by Dr. Andrew Weil, M.D., Pg 59

comparative studies investigating the impact of CR in humans are limited while studies on non-human species are more accessible. These species which have been studied include rhesus monkeys, lab rats, fish, and species of flies, along with a number of others. One of these studies, cited in *Science* magazine reported the following:

[From the **Abstract**] Restriction of caloric intake lowers steady-state levels of oxidative stress and damage, retards age-associated changes, and extends the maximum life-span in mammals.

**The caloric restriction model**

Although it has been known for about 60 years that a decrease in caloric intake by laboratory rats and mice, performed without malnutrition, extends the MLS [maximum life span], this phenomenon remained an underexplored curiosity until the mid-1970s. Notwithstanding, caloric restriction (CR) is now being increasingly used as a model regimen for understanding the basic mechanisms of aging, primarily because it causes an unambiguous, robust, and reproducible extension of MLS and delays many, although not all, age-associated biochemical, physiological, and behavioral changes. Life-span extension by CR has also been reported in fish, spiders, Daphnia (water-flea), and other nonrodent species, indicating a broad relation between energy intake and aging. [36]

There are multiple mechanisms involved with CR and a number of studies highlight on one or more of the following benefits of high quality life extension afforded to the participant: "behavior and learning, immune responses, gene expression, enzyme activities, hormonal action, glucose intolerance, DNA repair capacities, and rates of protein synthesis" all of which contribute to a "delayed aging profile." As the *Science* article points out, "Certain effects of CR in rats can be relatively swift", citing beneficial changes in the increase of *corticosterone* (in non-

---

[36] Oxidative Stress, Caloric Restriction, and Aging, by Rajindar S. Sohal, Rich Weindruch, from Science, July 1996, Vol. 273, Issue 5271, Pgs 59-63

human species this is the equivalent of cortisol, a critical hormone involved in regulation of energy, immune integrity, and stress responses) in the blood accompanied by as much as a 20% decline in blood glucose levels (blood sugar) within a week. Another key outcome was a corresponding reduction of blood insulin levels by as much as 50% within 3 weeks. "It appears that CR can rapidly affect the physiological state." [37]

One of these limited studies of caloric restriction in humans was published by Oxford University Press on behalf of the Gerontological Society of America in their publication *The Journal of Gerontology*, July 2015. That study, co-authored by some 22 researchers along with the CALERIE Study Group, was entitled **A 2-Year Randomized Controlled Trial of Human Caloric Restriction: Feasibility and Effects on Predictors of Health Span and Longevity**. It stated in part:

> **BACKGROUND**: Caloric restriction (CR), energy intake reduced below ad libitum (AL) intake, increases life span in many species. The implications for humans can be clarified by randomized controlled trials of CR.

> **RESULTS**: ...CR had larger decreases in cardiometabolic risk factors and in daily energy expenditure adjusted for weight change, without adverse effects on quality of life.

> **CONCLUSIONS**: Sustained CR is feasible in nonobese humans. The effects of the achieved CR on the correlates of human survival and disease risk factors suggest potential benefits for aging-related outcomes that could be elucidated by further human studies.

Other studies into the relationship between caloric restriction and cancer causation in humans are also quite valuable, revealing to those of us who, fearing the terror of such a diagnosis, what we can do to alter our lifestyle in order to prevent the disease. I cite the following:

> The specific relevance to humans of this caloric restriction is, as yet, undetermined. However, the inclusion in the human

---

[37] Ibid, Oxidative Stress, Caloric Restriction, and Aging, Science

diet of vegetables and fruits is associated with a decreased risk of cancer.

It is also known that caloric restriction can affect metabolic processes, including enzymes involved in carcinogen activation and inactivation. Reduced caloric intake also reduces the rate of cell proliferation or increases the rate of apoptosis (programmed cell death). Effects on cell proliferation appear to be a particularly significant means of modulating carcinogenesis, including effects on spontaneous tumors in rodents.

...Dietary restriction has enhanced apoptosis of preneoplastic cells, as well as decreased cell replication; these results suggest that food restriction may provide protection from carcinogens. [38]

As this excerpt states, (albeit in somewhat ambiguous language), a calorie-restricted yet highly nutritive diet *"may* provide protection from carcinogens." What we can firmly state is that this advantage of caloric restriction is not compatible or equivocal to the standard American diet (S.A.D.) which is overburdened with multiple compromises to the "eat less with higher nutrition" equation that makes for CR. The S.A.D. lifestyle has a heavy daily burden of excessive intake of junk calories. Recommendations from the Institute of Medicine for daily caloric levels range as high as 3000 for active males age 19-30. Yet still, the average American consumes as much as 25 percent more calories per day than U.S. Department of Agriculture recommendations. This is closely related to current historically high rates of overweight and obesity within this nation.

As well, caloric intake within the S.A.D. lifestyle has been rising dramatically, increasing some 20 percent between 1970 and 2010. As one article pointed out this transformation within this society:

---

[38] Carcinogens and Anticarcinogens in the Human Diet: A comparison of Naturally Occurring and Synthetic Substances, from the Committee on Comparative Toxicity of Naturally Occurring Carcinogens. The book examines numerous studies of the effect of caloric restriction on cancer-related processes.

**How Much You Need**

The average American adult woman needs between 1,800 and 2,400 calories per day, while the average American adult man needs between 2,400 and 3,000, according to the U.S. Department of Agriculture's 2010 Dietary Guidelines. Younger, more active folk can consume a higher number of calories and still maintain their weight. Eating just 250 more calories daily than your body requires for body functioning and exercise leads to a 26-pound weight gain in a year. A 20-ounce bottle of soda, half of a bakery cupcake and many fancy coffee drinks all contain at least 250 calories. [39]

How S.A.D. indeed is the average state of nutrition within the American population and, increasingly, other populations around the world are ever more eating like Americans.

How much more can be written that has not already been said about the negative impact that the so-called "Western Diet" has on the health outcome of modern societies? This Western Diet is often referred to specifically as the *Standard American Diet*, abbreviated as S.A.D. It has been proven in countless numbers of clinical studies that those who consume this dietary lifestyle run the risk of elevated rates of chronic diseases, including cardiovascular diseases, cancers, immune disorders and the entire spectrum of metabolic disorders (diabetes, obesity, high blood pressure, etc).

S.A.D. eating significantly increases the consumption of what are known as bad foods and doesn't include the healthiest foods in sufficient proportion to keep one disease-free. What makes this all the more problematic to the public is that the commercialization of food industries promotes marketing of many questionable food choices as being healthy when in actuality they are NOT compatible with the nuances of human biological nature.

American-style food is overloaded with sugar, denatured grain products, excessive fat, milk proteins, chemicals masquerading as foods

---

[39] The Average American Daily Caloric Intake, by Andrea Cespedes, Livestrong.com, May 2015

(preservatives, stabilizers, artificial flavors, and colors, etc.), acid-forming foods, improperly prepared foods, wicked food combinations, genetically-altered crops (often designed to tolerate high chemical loads) and is too often short on critical nutrients such as vitamins, essential fatty acids, fiber and more.

S.A.D. eating accompanies a caloric overload and the USDA has informed us that the Western diet has "nearly 1000 calories a day that can be directly attributed to added fats and sweeteners." This disruptive excess comprises more than one-third of the recommended average daily caloric intake for the non-athletic public.

The S.A.D. eater, contrary to virtually all advice on healthy nutrition, consumes far too little amounts of fresh vegetables and fruits which are proven to be the cornerstone of optimal nutrition. Many of us are eating too little of these necessary food categories while eating way too much refined grains, meat, sugar, canned soups, frozen foods, dairy and cheese, and artificial food ingredients. This all puts those who eat this way at greater risk of the spectrum of chronic diseases and disorders that shorten one's life expectancy as well as negatively impact one's chances of enjoying *healthy* maturation.

Another outcome of the S.A.D. eating lifestyle that we must consider is that who adhere to this dietary pattern also comprise the most drugged populations in the world. Prescribed medications associated with the S.A.D. life include anti-cholesterol agents intended to control elevated blood lipids, drugs to lower blood pressure and triglyceride levels, blood-sugar controlling agents, headache medicines, steroids for immune-related disorders, weight-reduction concoctions, anti-inflammatory agents, addictive opioid painkillers, as well as prescription and non-prescription analgesics to alleviate pain. [40]

CR also cuts down on the amount of acid-forming food one consumes. The human body functions best when the pH level of the blood is in the range of 7.25 to 7.45. Water has a neutral acid-alkaline balance of 7.0, so healthy humans need to be slightly alkaline. To do this properly, our

---

[40] 9 Charts that Show Why America is Fat, Sick & Tired, by Dr. Axe, from the website draxe.com

diet must avoid, as much as possible, an overabundance of *acid-forming* foods and promote the consumption of *alkaline-forming* foods.

It must be noted that not all acid-forming foods are bad for the human diet as there are some which contain wonderfully beneficial nutrients, such as citrus fruits, cranberry, and pomegranate. As well, there are different degrees to which foods create acidic conditions within the body, thus there are 1) very low acid forming foods, 2) low acid forming foods, 3) moderately acid-forming foods, and 4) highly acid forming foods. Depending on the starting points of those of us who wish to master a high-quality life extension, we can begin our transformation by eliminating the most undesirable highly acid-forming foods first and substituting more beneficial choices.

Extracted from an extensive listing of both alkaline and acid-forming foods published by *The Anti-Aging Newsletter*, some of the acid forming foods include:

### Moderately Acid Forming Foods

Nutmeg, coffee, casein, milk protein, cottage cheese, soy milk, pork, veal, bear, mussels, squid, chicken, maize, barley groats, corn, rye, oat bran, pistachio seeds, chestnut oil, lard, pecans, palm kernel oil, green peas, peanuts, snow peas, other legumes, garbanzo beans, cranberry, and pomegranate.

### Highly Acid Forming Foods

Tabletop sweeteners like (NutraSweet, Spoonful, Sweet 'N Low, Equal or Aspartame), pudding, jam, jelly, table salt (NaCl), beer, yeast, hops, malt, sugar, cocoa, white vinegar (acetic acid), processed cheese, ice cream, beef, lobster, pheasant, barley, cottonseed oil, hazelnuts, walnuts, brazil nuts, fried foods, soybean, and soft drinks, especially the cola type. To neutralize a glass of cola with a pH of 2.5, it would take 32 glasses of alkaline water with a pH of 10. [41]

S.A.D. eating, unfortunately, doesn't promote balanced consumption of the best alkaline forming foods. A simple rule to make our healthiest diet possible is to include several of the more alkaline forming foods as part of our daily consumption as well as to optimize the ways that these foods are produced. A baked sweet potato would be a wonderful alkaline forming choice but might be made far less beneficial slathered in butter or margarine. Some of the best choices, suggested by the *Anti-Aging Newsletter*, for alkaline forming foods include:

### Highly Alkaline Forming Foods

Baking soda, sea salt, mineral water, pumpkin seed, lentils, seaweed, onion, taro root, sea vegetables, lotus root, sweet potato, lime, lemons, nectarine, persimmon, raspberry, watermelon, tangerine, and pineapple.

### Moderately Alkaline Forming Foods

Apricots, spices, kombucha, unsulfured molasses, soy sauce, cashews, chestnuts, pepper, kohlrabi, parsnip, garlic, asparagus, kale, parsley, endive, arugula, mustard greens, ginger root, broccoli, grapefruit, cantaloupe, honeydew, citrus, olive, dewberry, carrots, loganberry, and mango.

As stated, this article on alkaline and acid-forming foods goes on in great length to point out the spectrum of choices we have in picking healthy foods to consume regularly. You will undoubtedly conclude that the common Western diet has been terribly imbalanced and that making sound corrections will allow one to enjoy more of the benefits of optimized nutrition toward healthy aging. The article summarizes the problem of *acidosis* with the following brief excerpt:

---

[41] Alkaline and Acid Forming Foods, from the Anti-Aging Newsletter, online at www.Anti-Aging-Today.org

An [overly] acidic balance will: decrease the body's ability to absorb minerals and other nutrients, decrease the energy production in the cells, decrease its ability to repair damaged cells, decrease its ability to detoxify heavy metals, make tumor cells thrive, and make it more susceptible to fatigue and illness.

The reason acidosis is more common in our society is mostly due to the typical American diet, which is far too high in acid producing animal products like meat, eggs, and dairy, and far too low in alkaline producing foods like fresh vegetables. Additionally, we eat acid producing processed foods like white flour and sugar and drink acid producing beverages like coffee and soft drinks. We use too many drugs, which are acid forming; and we use artificial chemical sweeteners like NutraSweet, Spoonful, Sweet 'N Low, Equal, or Aspartame, which are poison and extremely acid forming. One of the best things we can do to correct an overly acid body is to clean up the diet and lifestyle.

The ideas advanced in this chapter – numerous healthy benefits of caloric restriction, the negative impact of the Standard American Diet, as well as a focus on the worst offenders of S.A.D., acid-forming foods – will go a long way toward helping the individual and family to move firmly toward nutrition that complements our quest for longevity and healthy aging. Research confirms these findings is ubiquitous and can be verified virtually everywhere one looks for confirmation—*except* for within commercials for processed food.

The commercialization of the Western diet, failure of government regulatory agencies to curb this corruption, and the very culture of the S.A.D. lifestyle are all working together to produce skyrocketing rates of chronic disease and medical dependency. Correspondingly, there is skyrocketing investment in the industries of sickness, which, according to my perspective, should seriously be regarded as a national security threat.

How you will protect yourself, your family and friends is the most critical and controllable element within this broader nutrition equation. It is my absolute intention throughout this book to give you the best information and to arm you with tools, resources, healthy protocols and enough motivation to handle this serious task at hand as best as possible.

Longevity, along with healthy aging, is truly a blessing and a proper reward for our investments and efforts. Adapting our behaviors, adopting new habits and adjusting our diet to allow for caloric restriction to become an empowering tool, are all practical ways to make a big change for the long term. Take these tools and make them your own. Master each of them and be sure to spread this knowledge among all who would accept these gifts.

# Chapter 10 – **Women's Hormonal Health and Hormone-Balancing**

## Women React to Stressors

During this extensive study, we will frequently return to the central theme of *high-quality* life extension. How often have we heard it said that "a nation can only rise as high as its women"? Within this vision of mastering this spectrum of goals associated with quality living, the integrity of women's hormonal systems is a primary key to the successful outcome of health strategies within society.

In today's advanced technological societies, many women start to become affected by hormonal decay by the time they reach the age of thirty. This chapter explores factors which contribute to hormonal degradation, reveals critical insights and offers natural methods to slow down, arrest or even reverse this degeneration. Thus, if the suggested lifestyle changes are successful, women should realize a reduction in suffering from the spectrum of hormone-degenerative symptoms that include, pre-menstrual syndrome (PMS), menopause, infertility, reproductive disorders including various cancers, inflammation, uncontrollable weight gain, depression, osteoporosis and more.

As much as we search for and desire gender equality within civilized society regarding social, political, judicial and economic rights, when it comes to natural biology, there are significant differences between women and men which must be appreciated and, to the best of our abilities, managed appropriately. Among these are the different ways that the genders age and specific biomarkers that differentiate between men and women.

One such study, cited in the journal *Mechanisms of Aging and Development*, pointed out the differences in the manner of which the impact of redox biomarkers (products of the process of oxidation) affected brain changes in male and female rats that were specifically bred to resist obesity. The study looked at a spectrum of hormones related to mental functioning, glutathione (GHS), gamma-glutamylcysteine-synthetase (y-GCS), superoxide dismutase-1 (SOD) and a known protective enzyme called thioredoxin-1 (TRX-1), among other brain hormones. The researchers cited important findings which indicate that approaches toward men's or women's brain health might best utilize differing strategies. They said in part:

> Age-dependency of the markers differed between sexes, with SOD-1 and TRX-1 decreases out of hippocampus in females. Since antioxidants were reported to decrease with age in the brain of Wistar rats, maintenance of GSH levels and of protective enzymes mRNA levels in the LOU rat brain could contribute to the preservation of cognitive functions in old age. [42]

Those two conclusions are very important to both sexes, especially to women seeking to optimize brain and hormonal functioning later in life. The first suggests supplementation strategies to maintain glutathione levels as we age. Research indicates that there are well over a hundred thousand peer-reviewed scientific articles which have looked closely at glutathione (GHS), often referred to it as "The Mother of All Antioxidants." The proliferation of GHS deficiencies has been associated with premature aging, infections, chronic stress, injuries, GMO foods, artificial sweeteners, antibiotic overuse, and radiation exposure. [43]

The second suggestion in the previous excerpt is a bit more complicated as it relates to the maintenance of "protective enzymes mRNA levels", but we will herein simplify it. "Messenger RNA (mRNA) is a large family of RNA molecules that convey genetic information from DNA to the ribosome, where they specify the amino acid sequence of the protein products of gene expression." In simpler terms, it is a key factor in genetic expression into bioactive protein-based agents. Nearly all of the blueprints needed for life, of any living species, are encoded in the DNA mapping of the entire genome. RNA (ribonucleic acid) presents a pathway by which information is communicated to and from the DNA

---

[42] Gender-and region-dependent changes of redox biomarkers in the brain of successfully aging LOU/C rats, by Moyse, Arseneault, Gaudreau, Ferland, and Ramassamy / Mechanics of Aging and Development, July 2015, Vol. 149 19-30
[43] 9 Ways to Boost Glutathione, from Dr. Axe, from the website www.draxe.com

storehouse. RNA is involved in coding, decoding, regulation, and gene expression.

Protective enzymes are from the class of *metabolic enzymes*, manufactured by the body to regulate systemic functions. One important nutrient closely associated with this process is the mineral selenium. The impact of selenium deficiency in humans, as well as species used in laboratory experimentation, is well known within nutritional research. Symptoms of selenium deficiency can include low immunity, constant fatigue, brain fog and difficulty concentrating, reproductive disorders, hyperthyroidism, hair loss, fingernail discoloration, diarrhea, gastrointestinal problems, cirrhosis, and more.

Towards the aim of "maintenance of GSH levels and of protective enzymes mRNA levels" there is a spectrum of nutrition-associated solutions, which we will cover later in much greater depth. I do take a selenium supplement; if not daily, several times week.

## The Challenge of Hormonal Shifts with Aging

Among the many concerns that women have as they go through various stages of life are the broad array of effects that shifting hormones impose as the decades advance. Over the years attention has been paid to the impact of *estrogen* hormone levels in a woman's maturing body. One remedial strategy that has arrived and widely adopted, yet for which significant alarms continue to be raised, is *hormone replacement therapy (HRT)*. As our intention throughout the series of Living Superfood books is to approach our remedies in the most natural and least risky manner possible, I suggest that women thoroughly research HRT pros and cons before committing to synthetic hormone administration or any other therapies for which there are known risks.

To understand a bit more about what is involved with hormone replacement therapy, certain underlying facts must be considered. One such useful inquiry was published by *Life Extension Magazine*, entitled "Female Hormone Restoration: Estrogen Explained":

> To fully appreciate the complexity of HRT, it is important to understand the various forms of estrogen and their physiological effects. More than 15 forms of natural estrogen

have been identified (Taioli, 2010) including estrone, estradiol, and estriol.

Each of these estrogens has particular functions. Estradiol (E2) (the predominant form in non-pregnant, reproductive females) primarily aids in the cyclic release of eggs from the ovaries (i.e., ovulation). E2 has beneficial effects on the heart, bone, brain, and colon. Reduction in the level of E2 causes common menopausal symptoms such as hot flashes and night sweats. Estrone (E1), produced in the ovaries and fat cells, is the dominant estrogen in postmenopausal women. Estriol (E3) is secreted in large quantities by the placenta during pregnancy. However, it is a comparatively weak estrogen, and the form of estrogen least associated with hormone-related cancers. In Europe and Japan, E3 is frequently used for HRT (Head 1998; Kano 2002; Moskowitz 2006; Holtor 2009).

As noted in this excerpt, estradiol (E2) normally has "beneficial effects on the heart, bone, brain, and colon" while deficiency of this important estrogen hormone in maturing women is associated with the discomfort of menopause. And as the article pointed out, Estriol (E3), which is secreted in larger quantities during pregnancy, has been frequently used for HRT in Europe and Japan without the associated higher risk from other prescribed estrogen drugs.

In the U.S. some nine million women, nearly one-third of post-menopausal women, use the patented drug *Premarin* for hormone replacement therapy. Premarin is "made up of conjugated estrogens obtained from the urine of pregnant mares," hence the name **pregnant-mare-urine**. Manufactured by our national neighbor to the north:

Premarin is Canada's most lucrative pharmaceutical export to date. It is the most widely prescribed drug in the United States and holds 80% of the estrogen supplement market worldwide. ¶ Premarin was first marketed for menopause in 1942. By 1972, Premarin tablets were certified by the FDA as effective for treating menopause, and in 1986, based on studies conducted by Wyeth, the FDA approved Premarin for treatment of osteoporosis. [44]

## Dangers from Hormone Replacement Therapy

Estrogenic drugs are also being prescribed for women, as well as for men, to treat certain reproductive disease diagnoses, including cancer. This is particularly of concern since it is known that certain of the 15 different forms of estrogen are associated with *increased* risk of cancer growth. In addition, there is the notorious side effect of *chemical castration* when estrogenic compounds are prescribed to men undergoing prostate cancer chemotherapy; I regard this as a very sinister, dangerous and humiliating practice.

Noted side effects from Premarin usage in women include "stomach upset, nausea/vomiting, bloating, breast tenderness, headache, or weight changes" and patients are cautioned to be on the lookout for other serious side effects including "mental/mood changes (such as depression, memory loss), breast lumps, unusual vaginal bleeding..." [45]

To this list of precautions, the drug manufacturer's own website includes the following alarming warnings:

- Using estrogen-alone may increase your chance of getting cancer of the uterus (womb). Report any unusual vaginal bleeding right away while you are using PREMARIN. Vaginal bleeding after menopause may be a warning sign of cancer of the uterus (womb).

- Do not use estrogens with or without progestins to prevent heart disease, heart attacks, strokes or dementia (decline in brain function). ["Do not use...**with or without progestins**" – That is more than confusing, that is downright *frightening*!]

- Using estrogen-alone may increase your chances of getting strokes or blood clots. Using estrogens with progestins may increase your chances of getting heart attacks, strokes, breast cancer, or blood clots.

---

[44] Premarin—Facts & Opinions, from Project Aware, taken from the website of www.project-aware.org
[45] Premarin – Precautions, from WebMD, online at www.webmd.com

- Using estrogens, with or without progestins, may increase your chance of getting dementia, based on a study of women 65 years of age or older.

- You and your healthcare provider should talk regularly about whether you still need treatment. [46]

My suggestion is that any conversation you have with a healthcare provider that would prescribe such a dangerous and unnecessary concoction to you or anyone else starts off with the words, "WHAT IN THE HELL…"

### Bio-Identical Pregnenolone

Obviously, the symptoms of menopause and post-menopause are so disruptive to women that some solution must be brought forward. Fortunately, there are a number of beneficial foods, herbs, supplements and lifestyle modifications that can be utilized to serve the aim of high-quality life extension, thereby lessening the numerous disease risks associated with hormone replacement therapy. This brings us to the advantage of *bioidentical* HRT. Bioidentical hormones are considered by health advocates to be a "natural and safe alternative to standard hormone replacement therapy for menopause symptoms…" We can refer to an article entitled "**Is Bio-Identical Hormone Therapy Safe?**" published by *Everyday Health Magazine*. It read in part:

> Interest in bio-identical hormone therapy started to take off in 2002 when a large study called the Women's Health Initiative (WHI) was halted after researchers discovered an increased risk of breast cancer, heart attack, stroke, and other problems in post-menopausal women taking hormone replacement therapy.

> The hormone used in that trial was an FDA-approved combination of non-bio-identical estrogen and progesterone. Many women stopped taking hormone replacement therapy (HRT), and some went looking for alternatives.

---

[46] Premarin – Important Safety Information and Indications, from www.premarin.com

> Unlike conventional hormone therapy that uses synthetic hormones or animal-based hormones that are slightly different from a woman's own hormones, bio-identical hormones are biochemically the same as those made by the ovaries during a woman's reproductive years...[47]

Bioidentical pregnenolone supplementation has become more popular among women looking to alleviate the negative symptoms of hormonal maturation without assuming the numerous risks associated with other HRT therapies. According to several sources, pregnenolone, a glandular precursor, supports the body's natural production of hormones, promotes mental energy, reduces the impact of stress, supports brain function, increases the creation of new neurons, enhances memory and cognition, as well as helps alleviate suffering from chronic degenerative diseases such as Alzheimer's, Huntington's, ALS and Parkinson's.

An online nutritional supplement merchant shared the following about pregnenolone:

> Pregnenolone is found in larger quantities in the brain and cranial nerves than any of the sex compounds. Animal studies provide information showing the correlation between cognitive performance and the cerebral concentration of pregnenolone sulfate.

> With age, the amount of pregnenolone synthesized in the body decreases. Around age 75, it's believed to be reduced by as much as 60 percent (from the normal amount present at age 35).

As I furthered explored the practicality of using bioidentical HRT, focusing on the reported benefits of pregnenolone supplementation, I found more research which might be encouraging to women who want to alleviate these disruptive symptoms without increasing their risks of cancers and other chronic diseases associated with HRT therapies. One of these articles pointed out that bioidentical pregnenolone was produced from wild yams, grown in tropical regions:

---

[47] Is Bio-Identical Hormone Therapy Safe?, by Regina B. Wheeler and Kristen Stewart, Everyday Health online.

> Supplemental pregnenolone is molecularly identical to the pregnenolone that the body makes naturally. The raw material to create pregnenolone comes from wild yams (Dioscorea villosa), which are grown in Mexico and other tropical regions throughout the world. [48]

It should be noted that supplementation with natural pregnenolone is not only beneficial to women but to men as well. Keep in mind that pregnenolone is a precursor element used by the body to manufacture a spectrum of hormones. Still, its use for menopausal women cannot be understated. Wild yam has been studied extensively for its impact on women's health and an extract made from wild yam has long been shown to provide menopause symptom relief with a very low risk of side-effects. Wild yam extract is widely touted as a natural means of providing positive benefits for menopausal symptoms, normalizing blood lipids and for balancing sex hormones.

Dr. Edward Group, in an article entitled "**10 Best Herbs for Female Hormone Balance**" listed a number of herbs used throughout the world for alleviating symptoms of hormone decline attributed to maturation and menopause. He included noted remedies from the *Ayurveda* (an ancient nutritional healing system from India), along with localized solutions used in South America, China, the Caribbean, Europe, and Southern Asia. These are, as listed by Dr. Group: 1) Ashwagandha, 2) Avena Sativa, 3) Catuaba bark, 4) Epimedium (aka Horny Goat Weed), 5) Maca (root), 6) Muira puama, 7) Shilajit, 8) Suma, 9) Tongkat Ali, and 10) Tribulus Terrestris.

Of this list, many of us may be familiar with maca root, which has become somewhat popularized as a superfood and often referred to as "the Andes aphrodisiac." It is grown above 10,000 feet in the Andes Mountains of South America, where, among other uses there, farmers use it to restore fecundity to aging sheep.

Of the herb Tongkat Ali, the author notes:

> Tongkat Ali is consistently referred to as the greatest natural aphrodisiac known to man. Used in Malaysia by women to

---

[48] Ibid. Regina B. Wheeler

stimulate libido and increase the sensitivity of erogenous zones, Tongkat root also supports energy levels, cognitive function, and creates positive responses to stress. Researchers have found it boosts testosterone levels and promotes hormonal balance. [49]

Tongkat Ali is also marketed as a male enhancement supplement as "Men's Passion Booster."

Dr. Axe also has also posted online another article, "**10 Ways to Balance Hormones Naturally**" which focuses on supplements, foods, a critical analysis of cooking oils, inflammatory conditions, environmental stresses, toxic chemicals and other lifestyle factors which impact hormone balance. Food solutions include: 1) Eat coconut oil and avocados, 2) Supplement with adaptogen herbs, 3) Balance omega-3/6 ratio, 4) Heal leaky gut, 5) Eliminate toxic kitchen and body care products, 6) Interval exercise, 7) Get more sleep, 8) Limit caffeine, 9) Supplement with vitamin D3, and 10) Avoid using birth control pills. [50]

On the risks associated with birth control pills, Dr. Axe shared the following alarming points:

> I will keep on harping on this until birth control pills are banned. Just say no to birth control pills! In its simplest sense, "the pill" is hormone therapy that raises estrogen to such dangerous levels that it causes:

- Increased risk of breast cancer

- Increased risk of blood clotting, heart attack, and stroke

- Migraines

- Gallbladder disease

- Increased blood pressure

- Weight gain

---

[49] 10 Best Herbs for Female Hormone Balance, by Dr. Edward Group, from www.globalhealingcenter.com
[50] 10 Ways to Naturally Balance Hormones, from www.draxe.com

- Mood changes
- Nausea, irregular bleeding or spotting
- Benign liver tumors
- Breast tenderness

He closed the article by issuing a stern warning about the use of birth control pills: "I cannot urge you strongly enough to stop using them immediately. There are many other (safer) ways to prevent pregnancy." I hope that women will take this warning seriously and make sure that these dangers are communicated to younger women as well. Such avoidance of potential hormone stresses, implemented early in life, can likely have a tremendous impact on the quality of life well into advanced maturity.

We must summarize this chapter's focus on the special need for women of all ages to preserve their hormonal integrity and to achieve, as best as possible, high-quality life extension. Key lessons we have pointed out include the need for antioxidants, paying attention to the delicate balance of brain chemistry, the spectrum of estrogen hormones that make up a woman's complex biochemistry, stresses on the maturing glandular system, strategies for safe hormone replacement therapy, as well as herbs, supplements and foods that assist in natural rebalancing of biochemistry. Women, and the men who love them must comprehend the risks of certain commonly-practiced lifestyle habits that can have a serious negative impact on health outcome.

While the information that I studied during this particular inquiry into women's hormonal health could have a tsunami of detailed analysis, I trust that you will have gained sufficient insights within this chapter to allow you to seize the momentum and implement lifestyle modifications that will further your plan to enjoy both healthy maturation and extended longevity.

# Chapter 11 – **Superfood for Longevity: Full-Spectrum Hyper Nutrition**

## Dangers from the S.A.D. Diet

Let's begin this examination of a highly-idealized nutritional regimen by reminding the reader of the big problems associated with the Standard American Diet (S.A.D.), also known as the *Western Pattern Diet* or "the meat-sweet diet":

> The Western pattern diet, also called Western dietary pattern or the meat-sweet diet, is a dietary pattern originally identified through principal components analysis or factor analysis to identify commonly associated foods in the diets of several independent cohorts in the United States, with a very similar "Western" pattern also observed in a cohort of Australian adolescents. It is characterized by higher intakes of red and processed meat, butter, high-fat dairy products, eggs, refined grains, white potatoes and French fries, and high-sugar drinks. It is contrasted with a "prudent" diet found in the same populations, which has higher levels of fruits, vegetables, whole-grain foods, poultry and fish. [51]

This Wikipedia posting goes on to list several Western pattern diet-associated health concerns and risks:

> Compared to the "prudent" diet, the Western pattern diet, based on epidemiological studies of Westerners, is positively correlated with an elevated incidence of obesity, death from heart disease, cancer (especially colon cancer), and other "Western pattern diet"-related diseases. Breast cancer epidemiologists have found that women with a more Western

---

[51] Western pattern diet, from Wikipedia.com

diet have a nominally increased risk of breast cancer that is not statistically significant.

What the authors refer to as a "prudent diet" is still quite far from an "optimized diet" for our herbivore and fruitarian human physiology. Without going into minute details of why many of this culture's so-called "prudent" food choices are incompatible with our desire for optimal health, we must emphasize that the best nutrition for us is built upon a certain foundation, to include factors such as: plant-based, non-GMO, whole grains, fresh and organic, enzyme-rich (hence, as much as possible, uncooked), the least amount of processing, and avoidance of chemical flavors, sweeteners, preservatives or artificial colorings. Our approach is to focus our diet upon foods containing a broad spectrum of the critical nutrients which are necessary for all the body systems to have the raw materials for full functionality.

## How to achieve optimized nutrition

In my book *LIVING SUPERFOOD RESEARCH: Don't Get Sick, Stay Off Drugs and Live a Long Time*, Chapter 15 was entitled "Full-Spectrum Hyper Nutrition: Unleash Your Miracle." Within that chapter, I highlighted the critical importance of 6 classes of nutrients which we extract from our food. I have expanded and clarified that list in the 3 years since writing that chapter to eight critical categories of nutrients that make up the foundation of complete nutritional health; adding hydration and fiber to the list. These now eight categories encompass hydration, vitamins, minerals, enzymes, proteins/amino acids, essential fatty acids, carbohydrates, and fiber.

If our diet incorporates all eight of these nutrient classes – if they are consumed in as pristine form as possible and not compromised by chemicals masquerading as food, pesticide residues, endocrine-disrupting chemicals,  and other byproducts of the modern, industrialized food production system, and if they have not been overly compromised by cooking techniques—then we know our body will have sufficient raw materials for our various systems to function in the best manner for which they were designed. Regarding consuming this entire spectrum of critical nutrients, there is absolute truth to the cliché, "You are what you eat."

In the previous Superfood book, I shared extensive properties and benefits associated with each class of nutrients and herein I will only share brief excerpts on each of those we've previously cited. I hope that you will feel compelled to get the book **LIVING SUPERFOOD RESEARCH**, as it contains 20 chapters and 4 appendixes that are quite thorough on the research that supports vegan, raw, superfood, detoxification, and organic gardening lifestyles. So let's just briefly take a closer look at these 8 critical classes of nutrients.

1. **Hydration** – By the time that you are reading a book with this type of focus, you have obviously heard a lot of facts about how much water you should be drinking daily to optimize your health. Let's focus on some surprising facts linking water to longevity:

   a. At birth, a baby's body is made up of around 85% water, during healthy adulthood, this should average about 75% of body mass.

   b. People with chronic illness are usually dehydrated. This can amount to 65% hydration for men and as low as 52% for women.

   c. At the brink of death, hydration generally dips another 10% and severe dehydration is considered to the single greatest indicator of impending death.

   d. As one article put it: "Think of plants and leaves that are dead. They dry up and become brittle and fragile. Most people literally shrink and dry up as they age past a certain point (wrinkles, loss of height and muscle mass) due to severe chronic dehydration from not getting the benefits of drinking water daily." [52]

2. **Vitamins** – These critical nutrients can be broken down into two basic categories: water soluble and fat soluble. They are necessary for regulating metabolism and assisting the biochemical processes that release energy from digested food. Our need for vitamins is in minute quantities. Water-soluble vitamins must be taken daily and best obtained from fresh, whole food sources; they include vitamin C and the B complex vitamins (B1 thiamine, B2 riboflavin, B3 niacin, B5 pantothenic acid, B6 pyridoxine, B7 biotin, B9 folic acid, and B12).

---

[52] The Health Benefits of drinking water daily are innumerable., from Secrets of Longevity, www.secrets-of-longevity-in-humans.com

Fat or oil-soluble vitamins can be stored for longer periods of time, in the liver and fatty tissues of the body, and thus needn't necessarily be consumed constantly. Fat-soluble vitamins include vitamins A, D, E, and K.

3. **Minerals** – These are essential for cellular and muscle structure and are critical elements of blood, bone and nerve function as well. Minerals also function as coenzymes, enabling energy production, growth, and healing. "Bulk Minerals" (or macrominerals) are needed in large quantities because they form the basis of the major structures of the body, and include calcium, magnesium, sodium, potassium, and phosphorus; this is the same for humans as well as all plants and animals. "Trace Minerals" (microminerals) are needed in smaller amounts, yet are still vitally important for body function. The long list of trace minerals includes boron, chromium, copper, germanium, iodine, iron, manganese, molybdenum, selenium, silicon, sulfur, vanadium and zinc. For many people supplementation of these minerals is good advice because of the mineral-depleted foods too many of us rely upon for our basic nutrition. Yet the ideal way to access both bulk and trace minerals is through eating a whole food, plant-based diet as well as naturally exposing our skin to soil made up of these elements – we need to remember to play in the dirt from time to time.

4. **Enzymes** – Food enzymes function as activators, catalytic agents, allowing for molecules within our food to interact and form themselves into more complex chemical compounds or, conversely, break down complex chemicals into more basic molecules. They function in much of the same manner as heating food, stimulating the various vitamin and mineral elements to interact, and facilitating chemical formation. There are three types of enzymes within the body: metabolic enzymes, digestive enzymes, and food enzymes. One of the keys to obtaining the full benefit from food enzymes is to recognize the hard fact that naturally-occurring plant enzymes are largely destroyed by cooking. The rapid movement of molecules which takes place in heating the food neutralizes these valuable catalytic agents within fresh vegetables and fruits, where they are initially intended to help to break down decaying plant materials into their base protein and mineral components. When food enzymes

are compromised by processing, it requires the pancreas to work much harder to produce the replacement enzymes and other chemicals to complete digestion; the resulting stress can increase the weight of the pancreas by as much as 25%.

5. **Proteins/Amino acids** – Proteins are the basic building blocks of cellular life and amino acids, which are the building blocks of proteins, are the end product of protein digestion. These nutrients are critically necessary for forming cellular matter, tissue, muscle, body mass as well as structures within the body and brain. There are 23 different amino acids which are necessary for life, combining to create the proteins which comprise our molecular biology. These proteins then form into more complex tissues, organs, bones, and other structures. Of these 23 amino acids, 9 of them are considered *essential amino acids*, meaning that they are not only indispensable but, because they are not manufactured by the human body, must be obtained within the food we consume. While it is known that eating a diet inclusive of animal flesh can supply these 9 essential amino acids, vegetarians and vegans can gain access to adequate quantities of essential amino acids by eating a diet which includes a wide variety of nuts, seeds, whole grains, and legumes. The optimal way to get these essential nutrients within the plant food spectrum is to get them from whole foods, fresh, organic and raw.

Further, the advantage of consuming essential amino acids from plant-based sources is that it significantly reduces the potential risk of exposure to a wide range of damaging toxins known to be found within meat, dairy, eggs, and seafood, which too often are loaded with steroids, hormones, antibiotics, parasites, bacteria and pesticides. As well, meat, dairy, and eggs contain high amounts of LDL, the "bad cholesterol" which is causative of cardiovascular disease.

6. **Essential fatty acids** – EFAs are the fats which naturally occur in many of the foods we commonly consume and are not synthesized by the human body. There are two families of EFAs that need be obtained from the diet: Omega-3 and Omega-6. Omega-9 is another essential EFA yet it can be manufactured by the body. EFAs support the structure of various body systems including cardiovascular,

reproductive, immune and nervous systems. They are needed for cell manufacture and repair as well as the production of prostaglandins, which fight infection and inflammation as well as regulate body functions (i.e. heart rate, blood pressure, fertility, and immunity). Omega-6 and Omega-3 must be consumed in a proper ratio and most people living within the Western diet are deficient in Omega-3 by a significant factor. Good sources of EFAs include *raw* fish oils (heating destroys linolenic acid, from which one obtains Omega-6) or better yet, linolenic-rich oils such as safflower, grape seed, sunflower, sesame, flax, hemp, peanut, palm, and olive oils. The percentage of linoleic acid in safflower oil is 7.8 times higher than that found in olive oil. The top three sources of linoleic acid in oils are safflower, grape seed, and poppyseed. Other excellent food sources include flax seeds, walnuts, cloves, seafood, Romaine lettuce, spinach, kale, greens, squashes, mustard seeds, and soybeans. Soy is most often difficult to digest and should best be obtained organic, fermented, raw or sprouted. One cannot overemphasize the necessity of consuming EFAs primarily from plant sources and in sufficient amounts to obtain these essential fatty acids. They are as important as any of the other critical nutrients toward optimizing health and preventing disease.

7. **Carbohydrates** – The bulk of the fruits, nuts, seeds, and vegetables we eat are made up largely of carbohydrates. Carbohydrates are themselves storage systems for a spectrum of the aforementioned key nutrients. Some carbohydrates are small molecules, called monosaccharides, or they can be formed as large molecular complexes, called polysaccharides. The two most common monosaccharides are the simple sugars glucose and fructose. Complex carbohydrates are plant starches, cellulose, and glycogen. Glycogen is a glucose polymer (bond of smaller structures) which functions as stored energy within the structure of plants, correspondingly serving the same function within the liver and muscles of humans. Other notable points about carbohydrates include:

a. Carbohydrates are absolutely necessary for our energy formation;

   b. Carbs should form the greater percentage of our daily food intake of about 45% of calories in combination with 30% protein and 25% fat;

   c. Best sources of carbohydrates include whole grains, beans and legumes, fruits, vegetables (especially green and leafy varieties) and root crops. Within these four categories are a wide variety of foods that we can combine in infinite manners.

8. **Fiber** – While fiber is a subset of carbohydrates, research into the absolute benefit of consuming the right amount of fiber in the daily diet merits its expansion as another critical class of nutrients. The benefits of a fiber-rich diet are many and are consistently associated with much lower rates of all chronic disease, especially cancers of the stomach and bowels, as well as cardiovascular disease. Within our Living Superfood nutritional pattern, the amount of fiber that one might consume is likely as much as 500% or more than that gained from the Standard American Diet average of 15 grams of fiber daily.

To illustrate the great benefit of this large increase in daily fiber intake, let's examine the following facts extracted from studies considering the differential rates of fiber consumption in the Western diet compared to average fiber consumption in the diet of African populations.

Researchers from the University of Pittsburg and Imperial College London conducted a study within which they swapped the diets of African Americans and an equal number from the KwaZulu-Natal province in South Africa. [53] Certain study methods and key findings were critical:

> The scientists began by studying the diets of 20 African Americans from Pittsburgh and 20 rural Africans in KwaZulu-Natal in their homes. The African Americans ate two to three times more fat and animal protein than the rural Africans did, and far less dietary fibre. ¶The researchers then ran tests on the microbes living in the guts of the two groups. They found that the American and African diets were associated with very different populations of gut microbes. The rural Africans had

---

[53] Bowel cancer risk may be reduced by rural African diet, study finds, by Ian Sample, from The Guardian, Medical Research, April 2015.

more carbohydrate-fermenting bugs, and others that produced a chemical called butyrate. The Americans had more microbes that break down bile acids. Colonoscopies revealed polyps - which can sometimes mature into tumours - in nine of the Americans, but none of the rural Africans.

After determining these background biomarkers regarding the health status of these two groups of African genetic relatives who also shared a number of socioeconomic similarities within their host nations, researchers swapped the diets of African Americans and their Zulu cohorts. The outcome was quite dramatic with regard to the reversal of each group's risk factors for cancer and inflammatory disease.

The scientists next invited the two groups to stay at local centres, where their diets were switched over for a fortnight. Instead of their traditional high-fibre meals, the rural Africans consumed a high-fat, high-protein diet of sausages, hash browns, burgers and fries. Meanwhile, the African Americans switched to a low-fat, high-fibre diet including corn fritters, mango slices, bean soup and fish tacos. ¶At the end of the two weeks, the team from the University of Pittsburgh and Imperial College London found that the African Americans had less inflamed colons than before, and a reduction in biological markers for cancer. The only downside of the diet seemed to be an excess of wind.

While the African Americans seemed to fare better on the high-fibre meals, the rural Africans appeared to do worse on the western diet. Tests on material taken from their guts suggested that their risk of colon cancer had risen.

This research study was originally revealed in the journal *Nature Communications*, in an article entitled "**Fat, fibre and cancer risk in African Americans and rural Africans**", published April 28, 2015. The abstract of the peer-review article specifically emphasized the impact of increased or decreased fiber and fat as primary agents affecting chronic disease risk. The study authors stated:

We performed 2-week food exchanges in subjects from the same populations, where African Americans were fed a high-fibre, low-fat African-style diet and rural Africans a high-fat, low-fibre western-style diet, under close supervision. In comparison with their usual diets, the food changes resulted in remarkable reciprocal changes in mucosal biomarkers of cancer risk and in aspects of the microbiota and metabolome known to affect cancer risk, best illustrated by increased saccharolytic fermentation and butyrogenesis [glucose fermentation in the gut], and suppressed secondary bile acid synthesis in the African Americans. [54]

## Chapter Summary

As we should now clearly see through our examination of these 8 basic nutritional classes, there is a substantial body of reliable research which points to the tremendous benefits of plant-based whole-food nutrition toward the specific aim of healthy aging. The Miracle of Life relies upon our proper acquisition of these various nutrients and facilitating their incorporation into our diet in the most efficient manner possible.

Conscious eating habits and informed awareness of the food environment become essential to managing this complex set of requirements while, at the same time, we strive to make it all seem natural and uncomplicated. You will find in time that it is merely a shift in your consciousness toward the foods you eat that will serve to facilitate this transition. I hope you get a chance to savor the flavor of this transformation as much as me and other Living Superfood enthusiasts whom I regularly encounter. Awareness of your own healing miracle is outstanding. And when that miracle is tasty and revitalizing...well, it doesn't get any better than that, does it?

You have undoubtedly often heard the cliché, "You ARE what you eat." In actuality you are *much more* than what you eat—you are a product of how you think, play, who you associate with, how you engage your creativity and manifest your spiritual nature. Yet, when this statement is pronounced regarding these eight basic nutrient classes, we now have

---

[54] Fat, fibre and cancer risk in African Americans and rural Africans, Nature Communications 6, Article number: 6342 , Published 28 April 2015

hard facts at hand to prove the absolute truth of the phrase. Now we know what strategies and tactics are proving to work best toward guiding our lives along a pathway where the ultimate destination is healthy longevity.

# Chapter 12 – **Review of The Body Quantum, by Fred Wolf**

*"I speculate that healing is a quantum physical process that can be understood as a phase harmony of quantum waves. By being with each other, we enhance this harmony, just as two magnets provide more strength than each magnet separately. To be healed, separate parts of the body also must begin to respond to each other in phase harmony.*

*"Accordingly, illness is defined as vibrations of quantum waves out of harmony with each other. Using quantum physics as a basis, diseases, in addition, are seen as a game of probability modified by our own deepest thoughts and wishes. We become ill, we feel depressed. But which came first, the illness or the depression? In quantum physics the answer is not so simple. For the depression and the illness, in a certain sense, are the same thing."*
— Fred Alan Wolf [55]

In this chapter, we utilize one of our favorite *quantum sciences* books as source material to look at root causes of disease and disorder, peering beyond common concepts we have been taught by those who "practice" standard allopathic medicine. From a quantum science perspective, everything that manifests within our physical environment is ordered up as minute patterns reflective of the flow of universal energy. How might we come to terms with our own unconscious invitation to disorders or

---

[55] THE BODY QUANTUM: The New Physics of Body, Mind, and Health, by Fred Alan Wolf , Pgs 219-220

to disasters that disrupt our healthy lives? Is it possible that we "begin to die" from age 30 or even from the very moment of birth?

Throughout the course of this volume of Living Superfood research, we are encouraging our followers to expand their conceptual framework regarding currently-accepted beliefs about health, nutrition, the role of mind-body-spiritual processes in our lives, and other avenues of organizing toward a healthy *paradigm shift*. It is likely that very few of us give regular attention to matters of molecular and sub-atomic physics, quantum biomechanics or to ideas of transcending the *seemingly* mundane state of ordinary consciousness.

The book we have in hand for this chapter of study, **THE BODY QUANTUM: The New Physics of Body, Mind, and Health**, by physicist Fred Alan Wolf, will hopefully help to stretch and expand your conceptual framework on how to secure a healthy lifestyle. Understandably, this book is quite extensive and pushes beyond common thinking in many areas related to quantum comprehension of our minds, body systems, intracellular processes, physiological structural integrity, energy generation, and other topics. For the sake of brevity, we will be restricting our investigation, as best as possible, to two central topics: 1) the link between quantum physics and pathogenesis (disease causation), as well as 2) quantum means of triggering natural healing processes (also known as epigenetic healing).

Writing in the introduction to Dr. Wolf's book, Larry Dossey, M.D. shares the following informative insight:

> Our models of reality determine in very real ways what we can observe, what we perceive to be important, and what we decide to do about certain problems. Nowhere is it more important to realize this than in the world of medicine, where human suffering and human lives are at stake. We are learning that what we cannot conceptualize we cannot implement—and so our hands remain tied, therapeutically speaking, to the time-honored pillars of drugs and surgery,

and we are prevented by our mindless models from executing valuable therapies that rest on consciousness. [56]

We are extended the invitation to think outside of the mainstream medicine cabinet, so to say. Let us continue this exploration to point out a few key ideas on quantum physics, disease causation and epigenetic healing from Fred Alan Wolf's book. Hopefully, we can generate newly-expanded parameters for thinking, believing, acting and organizing new pathways toward optimized health and wellbeing.

One of the considerations that I frequently share during health and nutrition workshops is this profound insight into the sheer scale of cell proliferation. Outside of our conscious consideration, our autonomous body systems are engaging in some pretty awe-inspiring biological processes.

Every minute in every human body some 300 million cells die. If cells were not able to reproduce themselves through mitosis, every cell in the body would be dead in about 139 days. (The body contains 60 trillion cells. Divide that by 300 million cell deaths per minute, and you get 20,000 minutes. Divide that by 60 minutes per hour and then again by 24 hours per day, and you arrive at 139 days). [57]

The author then goes on to explain in significant detail the miraculous process by which the DNA within the nucleus of each cell begins to reproduce and divide itself during the processes by which cells replicate. These four phases, for which we don't have sufficient space herein to share detailed explanations, proceed without our *conscious* consideration, but rely on the quantum body's autonomous intelligence:

- **First stage—Prophase**: Chromosomes begin to condense, the cell's nucleus starts to fade, the spindle-like centriole, around which DNA is coiled, separates into two and the normal 46 pairs of chromosomes double to 92 pairs;

- **Second stage—Metaphase**: The nuclear membrane dissolves, the denser portions of the two centrioles with their chromosomes begin

---

[56] From the Foreword to The Body Quantum, written by Larry Dossey, M.D., Pt IX
[57] Ibid, Pg 98

to move toward opposite poles of the cellular fluid (cytoplasm), and an "equator" begins to form around the diameter of the splitting cell;

- **Third stage—Anaphase**: The newly formed chromosome poles completely separate and the cell elongates;

- **Fourth stage—Telophase**: The cell further stretches, a furrow appears around the diameter of the cell, nuclear membranes re-form around each chromosome group and the cell splits apart, now forming two twin cells. [58]

As we will explain later in more detail, this process of cell division gets even more complicated in cells specifically involved in sexual replication. In the sex process, DNA chromosomes (from two opposite gender members of the same species) form into four groups instead of two, each containing 23 chromosome pairs, with the female ovum forming only X-chromosome pairs, while the male sperm producing both X and Y-chromosome pairs. "Too much information" you might be thinking right now – but this is just a brief attempt to explain the complexity of life at the cellular level over which you really aren't required to devote any direct conscious thought. As well, who among us were aware that there was any real difference between *reproduction* and *sex*, both of which are models of *replication*?

In the section of the book called "The Mind-Body Interaction," the author goes on to articulate the complex interaction between external events, our sensory perception of external stimuli, intuitive and memory processing of these thoughts, and the myriad of ways that these thoughts frequently materialize in some part or parts of our physical self – in simpler terms, how thoughts become things, including diseases and disorders.

...In this way, we use our intuition to internally process momentum experienced in the outside world.

It is in this way that external experiences, words and physical forces are experienced bodily; they end up as interplay between intuition and sensation, and, for that reason, tend to localize at key body sites. A disruption in intuition surfaces

---

[58] Ibid, Pg 99

as a sensation felt in the body. We feel hurt when our spouse says "Good morning" in the wrong way; the normal flow of countless good mornings is disrupted by an inattentive greeting, and our bodies undergo wincing pain. [59]

Taking this concept further, Wolf correlates this to the depth of intimacies that are exchanged between the infant and its mother; within her, all trust, security, and facility for life is invested. Yet, Wolf points out, when certain of the responses the mother shows to the child communicate sensations of tension from within her intimacy, the child's responses to these conflicting feelings can have a lifelong impact on the child's wellbeing. "This could lead to several setbacks in our later life. As teenagers and adults, our skin could take on these wishes, and we could develop acne, shingles, even psoriasis."

Chapter seven of Wolf's book is entitled "Healing" and therein the author states one of his main theses regarding the relationships of disease and healing to quantum processes:

> Thus, to be healed is to be "made whole," at one with the universe. We all respond to a loving hand, a sympathetic heart. Sympathy is a rhythmic understanding – a vibration of two together in harmony and phase... ¶ Here again the body quantum comes to the rescue. I speculate that healing is a quantum physical process that can be understood as a phase harmony of quantum waves. By being with each other, we enhance this harmony just as two magnets provide more strength than each magnet separately. To be healed, separate parts of the body also must begin to respond to each other in phase harmony. ¶ Accordingly, illness is defined as vibrations of quantum waves out of harmony with each other.
>
> ...The physical body and the mental thought are correlated. Illness, then, is seen as a choice, perhaps unconscious, made by the invisible observer inside us all. And these choices are

---

[59] Ibid, Pg 218

governed by several factors, including the physical and mental condition of the body and mind. [60]

The author describes an experience during a long vacation where he himself set aside his disciplined routine of daily health habits of exercise, temperance regarding smoking and drinking, as well as keeping to writing and research work schedules. While he noted pangs of guilt for his slackening behavior, he did note that his feelings conflicted:

> I also ate more, slept and lounged more, drank, smoked. I read easy and light novels, and failed to write a single word for more than a month. I had a marvelous time! But I came back feeling out of shape, groggy, and a little guilty for having abused my body so much (even though I'd enjoyed it!)

Putting this deviation into the context of how our mentality is related to disease and disorder, he wrote:

> It seems that when I am in shape, I have little tolerance for abuse, but when I am not, I can withstand and, indeed, even enjoy much greater abuse. No wonder alcoholics enjoy alcohol so much, and two-pack-a-day smokers enjoy that fortieth cigarette just as much as the first one in the morning.

To be clear, despite the sense of pleasure one might derive from engaging in common activities which could be construed as tolerating abuse (alcohol, smoking, recreational drugs, greasy, salty, sweet and highly processed foods, sedentary lifestyle, etc.), there are a myriad of corrupting impacts that such behaviors will likely have on our long term well-being; we have confirmed this throughout this research. The point of insight that I am aiming for with these excerpts is that our conscious awareness and discipline for optimal health habits creates a refined environment within our finely-tuned bodies. When we are either unaware of such lifestyle disciplines or experience them but subsequently fall back from our disciplined habits, there are consequences to be expected which manifest as quantum energy patterns emanating from deep within the unconscious mind.

---

[60] Ibid, Pgs 219-220

As part of my own frequent outreaches into the community as health advocate, consultant and instructor, I frequently encounter people who claim, with a sense of insight, "I used to be a vegetarian (vegan or some other manner of healthy disciplined lifestyle)", to which I generally reply, in a leading manner, "That's great. Tell me how you felt when you were living that lifestyle." The response to my prompt is fairly consistent and predictable. I'll notice as their eyes seem to focus on some distant place as they begin to describe some generally positive experiences with their weight, energy, immune strength, and other vitality advantages. My next inquiry then draws out a comparison between those described advantages and what they are currently experiencing after turning away from the particular discipline that they had experienced. The snap back to current reality appears as somewhat a paradoxical letdown but most claim that they desire to return to that previous set of disciplines that had produced such positive outcome in the past.

In another section of the book, Wolf examines "Facts about Disease, Aging, and Death." Therein he first writes about the seemingly fixed state of the limit of *human lifespan* and the reality of *average life expectancy*. While medical and anthropological research has fixed possible human lifespan at a maximum of about 115 years, according to Wolf, average life expectancy has continued to grow as populations within developed nations benefit from advances in a spectrum of means to overcome early mortality.

People within rich, developed nations these days rarely die prematurely from *classical diseases* like diphtheria, measles, pneumonia, flu, smallpox, bacterial infections, STDs, tuberculosis, typhoid, and whooping cough. Breakthroughs in medical science, such as the introduction of antibiotics, along with hygienic procedures which produce clean water, waste disposal, increased nutrient access, and precise diagnostic technologies, have all combined to lower childhood mortality and lessen deaths from these classical diseases. As a direct consequence, average life expectancy continues to increase in virtually all societies in the world today.

He then compares classical disease mortality, which is in decline, to a corresponding rise in the rate of death from *quantum diseases* which have also been with humans for eons, to include some of the most common chronic disease killers of our era:

> I would like to suggest that diseases can be separated into two groups: the *classical mechanical*, curable by such modern antibacterial agents as penicillin, and the *quantum mechanical*, which are not so easily treated. These latter include, but are not limited to, viral infections, cancer, atherosclerosis, diabetes, and several others.
>
> The quantum mechanical diseases (QMD) are with us today as they were in earlier times. Medical treatment does not appear to be the best way to solve these current health problems. The major chronic or quantum mechanical diseases are the biggest health threats. And the best treatment today involves not medicinal but the prevention of factors that are likely to induce decreased vital capacity.[61]

Regarding the quantum connection to diseases, this concept of "vital capacity" is very significant toward our comprehension of the foundation of disease and disorder, and correspondingly, the pathway we would best take to set ourselves on the right course toward healthy longevity. Throughout this book, nearly all our instruction leads toward the goal of increasing *vital capacity*, which is manifest on all levels of our existence: molecular, cellular, organic and systemic, as well as the "Whole Being", which unifies mind, body and spirit. Vital capacity is the sum of the wellspring which we constantly dip into to assure that we are living fully in the moment and on the right pathway to sustaining health and vitality for decades to come.

Wolf goes on to further explain this concept of vital capacity:

> "Vital capacity" is a difficult term to define. It refers to such obvious health signs as the ability to take air into the lungs, hold your breath, and blow out a candle at a certain number of paces; the velocity with which your nerve cells conduct electrical signals; the basal-metabolic rate; kidney blood flow; and other vital body functions. As we age, these functions all exhibit declines...

---

[61] Ibid, Pg 223

> I believe that the decrease in vital capacity with age is connected directly to quantum physics and results from errors occurring at the level of molecular processes, such as the building of complex protein molecules. It is these errors that produce the decrease in vital capacity that we call growing old. [62]

As the author states, the idea of stretching our age limits beyond 100, 110 or even 115 years is something that captivates the attention of the science community as well as the general public. Yet, for most of us alive today, this appears not likely to occur. While I have made a strong case throughout this book that one could master the possibilities of high-quality life *extension*, we must equally emphasize the need to master the extension of *high-quality* life. This should have us celebrating each passing decade during our senior years without burdensome disease symptoms weighing down our day-to-day enjoyment of life or generating cellular and organic damage from chronic inflammatory processes. Much of the success we strive for is based upon our ability to feel good about how great we feel.

Through our study of *The Body Quantum* and "The New Physics of Body, Mind, and Health", one of the most important breakthrough lessons learned is our comprehension of the extent to which *the body has a mind of its own*.

We should well note how the author uses the special example of "spontaneous remission" from life-threatening disease as a basis to highlight the role of the body's innate healing consciousness to accomplish that which modern medicine often cannot match, even with its most sophisticated technologies. Further, modern scientific medicine often doesn't even comprehend this body-mind-spirit healing axis as a viable or reliable means by which one could obtain optimal health, healing, and even rejuvenation. The fact, in this case, is that both unconscious psychology and spirituality do have direct influence over the microbiology which might lie at the heart of disease; this is the heart of the new frontier of *epigenetics*. It should naturally follow that the more we understand about this epigenetic process, the more we should be able to willfully direct it.

---

[62] Ibid, Pgs 223-224

In the end, our striving to master the potential within quantum healing processes allows us a renewed sense of hope for a healthy future. Living Superfood is one of the greatest tools by which we can construct reliable bridges into this new era of our self-determining health reality. Here is where our oft-cited axiom that "food is Nature's most perfect medicine" can be complemented by facts:

> Thinking of ourselves as machines for a moment, reflect on the fact that we are the only machines that enjoy the refueling process! Eating is both a necessity and a great pleasure for those of us able to reap the benefits of our society. This body machine not only enjoys fueling itself, it also is capable of repairing itself. It can take the most complex forms of molecular life, such as are found in plants and animals, and rearrange them into new life forms. Not only does it rearrange them, it causes them to take part in the great adventure called evolution. And as we evolve, so do our protein molecules—our DNA and RNA. [63]

In the afterword to the book, "The Body Future", the author Fred Wolf envisions the day when our mastery of great quantum processes of the universe, which includes mastering our personalities, bodies, health, and lifespan, expands to the point where we can exert more conscious control over these intricate processes with simple power of will. He leaves us with an encouraging perspective on what the future holds for mankind's benevolent evolution:

> ...I expect that we will be able to change our bodies at will. I expect that with that gain in sensitivity and consciousness new messages will be received and our evolution will be speeded up so fast that it will make our heads spin. Perhaps we will be able to heal ourselves purely by thinking positively about ourselves. Perhaps we will be able to regenerate new limbs, increase our intelligence, and even live for 500 years or more.

---

[63] Ibid, Pg 283

If we can learn to live together as a species, we will not just survive this world, we will create it as well as other worlds beyond our present dreams. The intelligence of the body quantum is absolutely unlimited. [64]

With these points and so many others that author Fred Alan Wolf shares throughout *The Body Quantum*, I am in complete accord. Contrary to so many frightening conceptualizations of how the future of science, health, climate change, our symbiotic relationship to other Earth species and our management of the commons will evolve together, I remain convinced that knowledge and understanding is the balm by which our collective soul can be healed. There is plenty of space upon which we can all thrive on this beautiful and fruitful, water –covered, blue galactic pearl we call our home—Planet Earth.

---

[64] Ibid, Pg 285

# Chapter 13 –Superfoods for Seniors, Book Review

## Boost Memory and Brain Function

During many years of study beyond the month-long broadcast series which spawned this book, I have long investigated nutrition that supports healthy brain function for older persons as well as throughout all stages of life. What I'd discovered was a spectrum of remarkable "superfoods" that not only enhance learning and memory but have even been shown to actually *reverse* degenerative brain conditions such as memory loss, dementia, Alzheimer's and Parkinson's diseases. As I have done so often during these years, I herein share an extensive list of these brain food aids, especially focusing upon those which contribute to enhanced cognition, memory and learning. As a culinary artist, I know that these foods can all be prepared deliciously as they are utilized to protect us from toxic environmental stressors which cause degenerative disease.

Within this review, we can share insights from **Super Foods for Seniors**, published by The Editors of FC&A Medical Publishing. As I re-read it, I'm reminded why I so value this book and thus wanted to write a brief review for this book on longevity. Beyond brain and memory-enhancing nutrition, other sections of the book which deserve attention include insights into healing herbs, foods that keep the colon and lower digestive tract functioning optimally, maintaining female and male hormonal integrity with specific foods for each gender, and a number of other practical topics. But, for now, let's focus on brain foods that can be used to counter brain aging.

In the chapter on "Memory Savers", the authors introduce us to **24 foods to keep your mind sharp**, with the following insights:

> Research has shown that your brain does not have to slow down, and you can help prevent mental problems that often develop later in life, such as dementia and Alzheimer's disease. By exercising your mind as well as your body, you'll

be ahead of the game as you get older. Things like reading, doing puzzles, and inventing memory tricks are good ways to keep your mind sharp.

But don't forget to pay attention to what goes into your body as well as your mind. The food you eat really does affect your brain, and poor nutrition will put you at greater risk for memory problems. Foods like nuts and cold-water fish give you lots of omega-3 fatty acids, a form of unsaturated fat that helps improve your brain's performance. And a diet low in fat and calories and high in certain vitamins, like C, E, B6, and B12, has been shown to protect against Alzheimer's disease. Don't forget to drink a lot of liquids as well. Dehydration can also cause memory problems. [65]

Therefore let us embark upon a journey of understanding this list of "24 foods to keep your mind sharp," with a brief excerpt on each item.

1.  **Boost your recall with asparagus** – "The B vitamins folate, thiamin, B6, and B12 are all key players in better brain function... One cup of fresh asparagus takes care of 17 percent of your folate needs for the day and is a good source of other B vitamins as well."

2.  **Make mustard your condiment of choice**—"That bright color comes from the spice turmeric, which is full of phenolic compounds known as curcuminoids... Although scientists are not sure what causes Alzheimer's, they believe the protein beta-amyloid plays a large role because they have found excessive amounts, called plaques, in the brains of AD sufferers. Curcumin may block these plaques from forming as well as remove the amyloid plaque itself."

3.  **Protect brain health with almonds**—"They're packed with omega-3 fatty acids... the almond is a rich source of vitamin E, another memory enhancer. New research has found almonds also contain substances that are like cholinesterase inhibitors, which are drugs used to treat Alzheimer's."

4.  **Mend your mind with apricots**—"This fruit's golden-orange glow comes from the potent antioxidant beta carotene... [which]

---

[65] Super Foods for Seniors, from The Editors of FC&A Medical Publishing, pg 36

protects the brain by fighting these free-radical intruders, and preventing and repairing the harm they cause."

5. **Count on cantaloupe to help**—"It is full of vitamin C as well as beta carotene. Studies find that low blood levels of vitamin C can impair your memory and mental abilities."

6. **Grab an [organic] apple a day**—"This old standby has a potent antioxidant that appears to protect brain cells from free-radical damage... Quercetin may be the magic compound. In experiments with rats, researchers found that brain cells treated with this antioxidant, and then exposed to cell-damaging hydrogen peroxide, had significantly less damage than cells treated with vitamin C or not treated at all."

7. **Power up with blueberries**—"You can reverse the effects of aging and keep your mind sharp. Do it all with sweet, delicious blueberries. The antioxidants in this deep blue fruit safeguard your brain against free radicals. They appear to slow – and even reverse – memory loss caused by free-radical damage."

8. **Take advantage of boiled rice**—"You lose electrolytes when you become dehydrated, and that can cause other serious problems as well. You need these salts and minerals in your blood, tissue fluids, and cells... Just cook up some rice, and drink the cooled water left in the pot." [I recommend using wild rice or brown rice as white rice has had much of its most important nutrients stripped away.]

9. **Stave off memory loss with olive oil**—"That's because of its omega-3 fatty acids, which boost your brain function as well as protect you against other health problems like heart disease and diabetes... Olive oil's 'good' fat molecules appear to buffer your brain against memory loss by patching up fatty membranes affected by aging."

10. **Enjoy a banana for a B6 boost**—"If you don't get enough of this important B vitamin, your brain may have a more difficult time making neurotransmitters, the chemicals that carry nerve impulses from cells to your brain. This can lead to depression, shortened attention span, and other problems. Studies have shown that people with B deficiencies score lower on memory and problem-solving tests."

11. **Prevent "mental meltdown" with amazin' raisins**—"These tiny fruits are packed with boron, a trace mineral the government doesn't consider 'essential,' but actually affects everything from hand-eye coordination to long and short-term memory."

12. **Sample seaweed for something different**—"They are loaded with vitamin B12, an important nutrient in maintaining memory... Many older adults are deficient in this vitamin, and up to 90 percent who lack B12 may develop memory loss or depression."

13. **Don't turn up your nose at turnip greens**—"Keeping your brain sharp at 70 may be as simple as eating vegetables like turnip greens and spinach, which are chock full of this potent antioxidant [vitamin E]. Vitamin E helps fight free radicals – unstable molecules that damage your cells. This damage has been linked to cancer, heart disease, and more recently, memory loss and Alzheimer's... So focus on getting your vitamin E naturally for the most benefit."

14. **Enrich your diet with spinach**—"You may have an underactive thyroid causing you problems. Nutrients like vitamins A, E, and D will keep your thyroid healthy and your mind sharp... Steaming is the best cooking method – even better than microwaving – for preserving the vitamins you need" [I recommend eating greens raw as much as possible to preserve the natural plant enzymes as well as critical nutrients which are damaged by cooking.]

15. **Try an egg-ceptional source of choline**—"Your body needs this nutrient to make acetylcholine, a neurotransmitter important for learning and memory... Egg yolks are high in cholesterol, too, and you don't want to add more from fatty meats and dairy." [Egg yolks contain the LDL or bad cholesterol which is something we constantly raise the alarm throughout this Living Superfood research. Plant-based sources of choline include Brewer's yeast, soy products, cauliflower, spinach, wheat germ, kidney beans, quinoa, rice, and nuts. [66]]

16. **Start with barley for breakfast**—"...according to a Canadian Study. Subjects began their day with cooked barley and enjoyed a boost in

---

[66] Rich Choline Foods and List of Vegan/Vegetarian Sources, from the staff of Nootriment.com

both memory and IQ test scores. Barley's secret to this morning miracle is energy from carbohydrates."

17. **Fight Father Time with the humble prune**—"Research shows it can help stave off the diseases of aging, including Alzheimer's and Parkinson's disease. Free-radical fighting antioxidants appear to be the key... Researchers in Boston have measured and studied antioxidants in foods and assigned them a score called the Oxygen Radical Absorbance Capacity (ORAC). Prunes registered a whopping 5,770 ORAC per 3 ½ ounce serving – more than twice as many antioxidants as the next highest food, its wrinkled cousin the raisin."

18. **Go "fish" for brain protection**—"...people who ate one or more servings of fish per week reduced their mental decline by 10 to 13 percent per year – the equivalent of being three to four years younger... previous studies have shown omega-3 may protect against more serious mental decline like Alzheimer's disease." [For vegetarians/vegans, excellent sources of omega-3 fatty acid include: flax, chia, hemp, sunflower and pumpkin seeds, leafy greens, mung, navy, kidney and soy beans, cabbage, winter squash as well as walnuts and pecans. [67]]

19. **Make a pot of lentil soup**—"A cup of lentils has 2.5 milligrams of iron, more than 25 percent of your daily requirement if you're over 50. Plus they're packed with healthy fiber...enjoy several bowls throughout the week to keep your iron levels up and your mind sharp."

20. **Cure memory loss with cabbage**—"Another fatty acid, phosphatidylserine (PS), may also give your brain a boost. It's a phospholipid, a fatty acid that is involved in communication between cells. Scientists believe as you get older your nerve cell membranes become less fluid and have trouble transmitting electrical impulses. This is one reason older people have more problems with memory and reasoning... Several studies have shown that PS improves memory and concentration and also relieves depression and stress."

---

[67] Plant-Based Foods With the Highest Omega-3 Fatty Acids, by Jonathon Engels, One Green Planet online, Sept. 3, 2014

21. **Get into the habit of drinking green tea**—"It may help protect your brain from the memory-robbing effects of amyloid plaque, a marker for Alzheimer's disease." [As well, green tea is an excellent source of antioxidants and other micronutrients.]

22. **Jolt your memory with java**—"Caffeine appears to stimulate the areas of the brain involved with attention and short-term memory... Too much caffeine can result in other problems, and researchers are not sure how it affects long term memory." [I quit drinking coffee completely when I came across research linking coffee to acrylamide (acrylic amide) and its associated carcinogenic effect in the body.]

23. **Try new recipes with ricotta cheese**—"Calcium plays an important role in the connections between brain cells. When you learn and remember something, calcium appears to set off chemical reactions that change connections between the neurons. This complex process is believed to be the basis of memory, learning, and brain development... Cheese is a good source of this vital nutrient, with part-skim ricotta a shining star at 669 milligrams per cup." [Those who choose only plant-based sources for this critical nutrient can source calcium from kale, collards, blackstrap molasses, tempeh, turnip greens, hemp milk, tahini, almond butter, beans, soybeans, broccoli, raw fennel, blackberries, black currants, oranges, apricots, figs, dates, artichoke, sesame seeds and amaranth. [68]]

24. **Relax with a glass of red wine**—"Wine has long been touted for its heart-healthy benefits, but recent research shows it may help your memory as well. Resveratrol, a compound found in grapes and red wine, appears to lower the levels of beta-amyloid proteins in the brain that cause the telltale plaques of Alzheimer's disease... If you enjoy a glass of wine now and then, choose a red variety made with Pinot Noir grapes to reap the most resveratrol."

I do have reservations about the suggestion that drinking wine is beneficial to brain health, as well as overall wellbeing. While I've always tried to be tolerant of other's desire to consume alcoholic beverages, including beer and wine, my own direction in life excluded all alcoholic

---

[68] 25 Vegan Sources for Calcium, by Becky Striepe, from Care2.com

spirits over 30 years ago. Contrary to the touted health advantages of moderate drinking, alcohol has been associated with several types of cancer of the mouth, larynx, esophagus, colon, liver, and breast as well as possible links to pancreatic and lung cancer. I prefer to just eat dark grapes for the very resveratrol nutrient that is the touted benefit of dark-colored wines.

Looking through this long list of "super foods for seniors" that specifically focus on strengthening brain function, memory, and nervous system integrity, I really can appreciate the advice that this editorial staff has compiled. Surely there were areas where my personal philosophy of the raw vegan diverged and I tried my best to point out key areas for each of us to be alert and, hopefully, do further research.

This is just a small section of the larger book which focuses on more than two dozen areas of our whole-body health where nutrition will positively assist our healthy-aging strategies. I can suggest without hesitation that this book *Super Foods for Seniors* should be in your health library.

# Chapter 14 – My Anti-Aging Arsenal of Supplements

## Are Nutritional Supplements Really Helpful?

People who come within my circle often ask me what I think of supplements. There are some public health advocates who have written or otherwise promoted the idea that supplements, vitamins, minerals, and others, are unnecessary and essentially amount to "expensive poop" when they are passed through the digestive tract without significant absorption. I have investigated this idea and cannot disagree that a significant proportion of the vitamins which are being sold are not particularly useful. Many commercially-promoted supplements contain chemical, non-organic and metalized-mineral substances that make them unnatural and incompatible with human digestion. Children's vitamins are one particularly suspicious category, where some of the ingredients are highly questionable. The most popular advertised brands of children's vitamins contain artificial sweeteners, artificial colors and animal-based gelatins. [69]

Still, within my own nutrition routine, I have and continue to use as many as 33 different supplements, above and beyond my daily regime of Living Superfood, which itself is among the most concentrated spectrum of nutrients one could imagine. When people ask me why I take supplements on top of Living Superfood, I share a few reasons:

- Because it is so difficult to buy 100% organically grown produce, some of that which is commercially available is grown in soil that itself is not as rich in minerals as would be ideal;

- Food is often shipped long distances between harvest and consumption, such as out-of-season crops from other countries or tropical crops. As such, picking fruit before it is ripe, along with other

---

[69] The Big Problem with Children's Vitamins and Supplements, by Carolina Buja, Newsweek, June 2015

transportation storage methods, can rob these foods of critical nutrients, especially water-soluble vitamins;

- As our bodies mature, our endocrine system ages (endocrino-senescence) and will produce lesser amounts of certain hormones that were abundant during the younger years. Supplementation with hormone rejuvenators is thus advantageous;

- The level of environmental stressors that we encounter today is the greatest that it has been in the history of our biological evolution and thus any additional support to bolster the antioxidants that counter oxidative stress serves greatly to our advantage;

- During our seasonal health-maintenance strategies, detoxification is one of the most valuable practices one can adopt. There are several detoxifying supplements which are helpful to maintain youthfulness.

For these and other reasons, I have dozens of supplements that I've added to my Living Superfood arsenal over the years. Herein I share my supplement secrets, supplying a few notes about each. For the following insights, I draw from a few books within my health reference library. I've also scoured the Internet to update my information base to explain my personal choices in supplements. Among the books I frequently utilize are included (but most certainly are not limited to):

1. REVERSE THE AGING PROCESS NATURALLY: How to Build the Immune System with Antioxidants—the Super-nutrients of the Nineties – Gary Null and Martin Feldman, M.D.

2. POWER AGING: The Revolutionary Program to Control the Symptoms of Aging Naturally – Gary Null, Ph.D.

3. MIND POWER: Rejuvenate Your Brain and Memory Naturally – Gary Null, Ph.D.

4. THE LONGEVITY BIBLE: 8 Essential Strategies for Keeping Your Mind Sharp and Your Body Young – Gary Small, M.D.

5. HEALTHY AGING: A Lifelong Guide to Your Physical and Spiritual Well-Being – Andrew Weil, M.D.

6. STOPPING THE CLOCK: Longevity for the New Millennium – Dr. Ronald Klatz and Dr. Robert Goldman

7.   LIFE EXTENSION MAGAZINE – Available by subscription in print and online at LifeExtension.com

The following list of nutritional supplements is currently in my vitamin, mineral and herbal stash as of the spring of 2016.  It is quite extensive, yet I have other supplements on my shopping list that I plan to acquire soon.  This list does not cover culinary herbs which also have such powerful health-promoting effects that they are used as often as possible in food preparation, such as turmeric, ginger, garlic, cinnamon, cayenne pepper, coconut oil, nutritional yeast, etc.

1.   **Acetyl L-Carnitine HCl** – Increases cellular energy, enhancing mood, alleviating nerve pain, promotes growth of nerve cells, prevents death of brain cells, combats amyloid beta peptide (plaque) in Alzheimer's, reverses mild cognitive decline, averting and managing depression, mental fatigue, physical fatigue, useful for MS disease symptoms, chronic fatigue syndrome, various cardiovascular effects, increased blood flow, supports heart muscle recovery following a heart attack (myocardial infarction), prevents ischemia (lack of blood flow and related tissue damage), good for skeletal muscle health, reversing erectile dysfunction, and halting brain aging.

2.   **Activated Charcoal** – This detoxifying dietary supplement has a multitude of uses for those who try to avoid damage from environmental, commercial and chemical toxicants.  Specifically, as an anti-aging agent, it helps prevent cellular damage to the liver and kidneys, supports strong adrenal glands, and removes toxins that can cause oxidative stress damage.  It is used to trap toxins and chemicals in the body, allowing them to be eliminated through the bowels.  As well, in emergency centers, AC is used to treat acute poisoning and drug overdoses.  It is also known to reduce gaseous bloating, lower the bad (LDL) while increasing the good (HDL) cholesterol, manage bile flow during pregnancy, relieve migraine headaches, and even prevent alcoholic hangovers.  Powdered activated charcoal is also touted as a teeth whitener as well as other oral benefits such as preventing cavities, bad breath, and gum disease.  AC is an important component of water filters, removing fluoride, and can be used for various skin conditions including insect bites, rashes from plant toxins and even snake bites.  Taking activated charcoal after eating non-organic fruits and vegetables is a great way to help to neutralize

any effect of pesticide and chemical residues in these foods. For those who are on prescription drugs, caution is recommended as activated charcoal is very likely to interact with a spectrum of pharmaceutical drugs; therefore, you should consult with the prescribing physician before beginning an AC regimen.

3. **Alpha Lipoic Acid** – A natural cofactor for mitochondrial enzymes, ALA breaks down fatty acids, enhances cellular energy, is a potent antioxidant, increases intracellular levels of vitamin C and glutathione, anti-aging properties, and protecting brain cells from oxidative damage. ALA decreases insulin resistance while building the body's antioxidant defenses. It is also recommended to those diagnosed with metabolic syndrome (described in Chapter 3) or who might be susceptible to obesity or type-2 diabetes.

4. **Ashwagandha** – This is one of the world's oldest, most researched and powerful adaptogen herbs, and is considered one of the most effective anti-aging supplements one can incorporate. With a record of as many as 3000 years of usage in India, Africa, and Western Asia, the many benefits of Ashwagandha (also known as *Withania somnifera*, *Indian ginseng* or *winter cherry*) are widespread and quite renowned. Validated benefits include: boosting thyroid glandular function (hypothyroidism), neuroprotective, effective against anxiety and depression, anti-inflammatory, strengthens adrenal gland function, insomnia relief, combatting mental stresses and reduces cortisol levels, balances blood sugar, fighting or preventing cancer and tumor formation, reduces brain cell degradation, improves memory, boosts immune system function, increases stamina, muscle strength and endurance, improves sexual desire, function and fertility, a powerful antioxidant, contains a spectrum of amino acids (including tryptophan), lowers cholesterol and triglycerides, supports cardiometabolic health, and even more.

**WebMD** states that "Ashwagandha is used for arthritis, anxiety, bipolar disorder, attention deficit hyperactivity disorder (ADHD), balance, obsessive-compulsive disorder (OCD), trouble sleeping (insomnia), tumors, tuberculosis, asthma, a skin condition marked by white patchiness (leukoderma), bronchitis, backache, fibromyalgia, menstrual problems, hiccups, Parkinson's disease, and chronic liver disease. It is also used to reduce the side effects of medications used to treat cancer and schizophrenia. Ashwagandha is used to reduce levels of fat and sugar in the blood. Ashwagandha is also used as an 'adaptogen' to help the body cope with daily stress, and as a general tonic." Applied as a topical ointment, Ashwagandha is applied for treating wounds, backache, and one-sided paralysis (hemiplegia).

5. **Astragalus** – A wonderfully useful adaptogen that is particularly valuable for boosting the immune system. Astragalus has a long history in Chinese medicine and recent research confirms the antiviral and immune-enhancing properties of the root, recommended to people with weakened immunity or who might be undergoing immune-suppressing cancer chemotherapy.

6. **Bentonite Clay** – One of my favorite cleansing agents that I use during seasonal detoxification. Bentonite clay has a long tradition as a healing agent, affecting such conditions as gaseous bloating, constipation, irritable bowel syndrome, protecting the immune system and binding to toxins in the digestive tract, thus allowing these bound toxins to be quickly eliminated. Its benefits include removing fluoride residue from fluoridated water supplies, as well as fighting volatile organic compounds (VOCs) from the tremendous spectrum of chemical exposures we encounter in cleaning supplies, industrial chemicals, building materials and literally hundreds of other daily exposures. The clay also helps in chelating the body of toxic metals such as mercury, cadmium, lead and toxic chemicals such as benzene. Because of its role in ridding the body of such a broad spectrum of free radical generating toxins, its use is a good supportive agent toward maintaining a strong immune system. For people who eat meat, bentonite clay is highly recommended for combating the high amount of CAFO-encountered toxins known to be found in the meat, many of these, including aflatoxins found in poultry feed, are directly associated with increased risk of cancer.

7. **Cascara Sagrada** – A favorite colon cleansing supplement, it is also known as bitter bark, buckthorn, sacred bark (cascara sagrada translated into Spanish), purshianae, and chittem bark. While its colon cleansing, constipation relieving and other gastric-distress-relieving properties are notorious, including treating or preventing gallstones, herbal compounds containing sacred bark have many

benefits. These include: fighting symptoms of aging such as wrinkles, blemishes, acne and patchy skin as it also helps the skin to remain hydrated; promotes healthy hair and combats dandruff and lice on the scalp; as well can be used to treat insomnia, aid in weight loss (without some of the notorious side effects of common weight loss supplements); and because of its high level of anti-oxidants, helps to treat and prevent cancer. Sustained and frequent usage is discouraged because it can cause diarrhea as well as a dependency on the herb. Pregnant and lactating women are discouraged from using cascara sagrada and prolonged use of this herb without taking a pause may be associated with potassium loss from the body.

8. **CoQ10** – A mitochondrial energizer, counters heart ailments and neurological disorders, is a cancer-fighting agent, prevents migraine headaches, slows macular degeneration, slows the progress of neurodegenerative diseases (Parkinson's, Alzheimer's, ALS and others), protects against hearing loss, improves cognitive function, extends life span, assists muscle regeneration, good for post-surgery recovery, preserves male fertility, fights amyloid beta peptides (Alzheimer's associated plaque in brain tissues), supports diabetes treatment, lowers blood triglycerides, and counters the effects of chemotherapy.

9. **DHEA (dehydroepiandrosterone)** – Is a hormone naturally produced in the body that has come to be one of the most popular hormonal supplements on the markets. DHEA levels begin to decline for most adults in the mid-30's. Supplementation with this powerful hormone can get athletes banned from competition if it shows up in elevated levels during athletic drug testing. Despite the ban, DHEA has proven to offer great health benefits and very low risk to the user when used moderately. Reported benefits of supplementing with dehydroepiandrosterone include (but are not limited to): combatting depression, obesity, adrenal fatigue and Addison's disease (insufficient steroid hormone production), autoimmune diseases (lupus, multiple sclerosis, and chronic fatigue syndrome), osteoporosis, sexual disorders including erectile dysfunction and vaginal atrophy, improving sexual desire, performance and satisfaction, psychological conditions including schizophrenia, anorexia, enhancing mood and memory, type 2 diabetes,

combatting all-cause morbidity (premature death of all causes), boosting energy, increasing bone and muscle strength, promoting nerve cell growth, combatting systemic inflammation, prolonging cell longevity and slowing signs of aging by increasing collagen formation, shielding neurons from toxic stressors, post-stroke recovery, improving skin integrity, combatting insomnia, as well as balancing production of the major male and female hormones testosterone and estrogen. For so many reasons, DHEA is considered one of the most powerful and effective anti-aging supplements one can include in their arsenal.

10. **EDTA** – EthyleneDiamine TetraAcetic Acid is a synthetic amino acid which is related to vinegar. It was developed in the 1930s to reverse heavy-metal poisoning from ingesting lead, mercury, aluminum, cadmium, arsenic, and excessive iron. Because EDTA can also negatively impact serum levels of key electrolytes, it is recommended that you access forms of this chelation agent which also are fortified with minerals (calcium, di-sodium). The form I use is encapsulated, while severe, acute poisoning with heavy metals is treated intravenously by emergency medical technicians. While I have used EDTA along with bentonite clay, herbal laxative, aloe vera and other detoxification agents quarterly for over a dozen years, I do recommend you study this powerful agent before committing yourself to a regimen; sometimes the mass of toxins which are pulled from the blood can be a bit overwhelming, resulting in nausea, vomiting, and diarrhea. Successful administration of chelation therapy can seemingly take years off one's sense of aging within just a few days. Benefits of EDTA chelation can include relieving symptoms of cardiovascular injury (including heart attack and stroke as late as two years after the event), treatment of senility, dementia and Alzheimer's, reducing high blood pressure, reversing diabetic gangrene thus preventing the need for lower extremity amputations, improving memory, normalizing heart arrhythmia, reversing calcification of body organs, as well as preventing or reversing osteoarthritis.

11. **Eleuthero (Siberian Ginseng)** – Highly touted as one of the most valuable herbal supplements, this powerful herb has a long record of use within Chinese medicine. Its many useful applications include

speeding cold relief, aids in mental performance, fights stress-related fatigue, successful management of osteoarthritis, fights oxidative stress, lowers cholesterol levels in the blood, blocks the impact of adrenal cortex in stress responses, boosts immune function, combats inflammation promotes liver health, is good for the circulatory system, enhances memory alertness and concentration, increases blood flow to the brain, balances hormones affecting mood, contributes to a healthy endocrine system, prevents impotence, improves symptoms of menstrual disorders, and is useful for treating insomnia and nerve-related mental disorders.

12. **Eyebright (Euphrasia Officinalis**) – This herbal remedy has a long record in natural treatments for eye conditions, infections and irritations such as conjunctivitis (pink eye), other systemic inflammatory conditions, treatment for colds and allergies, as well as hepatoprotective benefits (blood, circulatory and liver protective), and enhancing memory due to flavonoids and beta-carotene constituents of the herb. As we age, the strength of our eyesight can be impacted by several factors, including the weakening of our immune system. The combination of flavonoids (highly beneficial plant-based metabolites), tannins (natural organic molecules with a spectrum of benefits related to protein metabolism and the regulation of amino acids and alkaloids), and iridoid glycosides (needed for digestive processes, laxative, and antimicrobial functions) – all make eyebright a wonderful anti-aging supplement.

13. **Ginko Biloba** – Good when combined with Panax Ginseng, Ginko Biloba is useful for reinforcing mental faculties, memory improvement and vision, increased vascular dilation, while combating depression, headache, sinusitis, vertigo, tinnitus, anti-oxidant, reduce blood viscosity, macular degradation, Alzheimer's, cerebral atherosclerosis, dementia, menopause, retinopathy, impotency, Parkinson's, diabetes-related nerve damage and poor circulation, allergies, vertigo, leg cramps and PMS. It is thought to work in a large part by inhibiting oxidative cell damage and improving cerebral circulation as well as other circulatory issues throughout the body.

14. **Joint Support (Glucosamine, MSM & Chondroitin**) – This combination is directed at cartilage sites throughout the body,

especially the joints. It serves to relieve inflammatory conditions, arthritis and to slow joint deterioration.

15. **Lutein** – Found naturally as a yellow-pigment carotenoid in many fruits and vegetables, lutein functions as an antioxidant protecting against the damage of free radicals. Not manufactured by the body, it must be obtained from food or supplements. Other benefits include eye health, resisting macular degeneration (the leading cause of blindness in older adults), cataracts and retinitis pigmentosa. Additionally, because of the powerful antioxidant effects of beta-carotene, lutein is believed useful in the prevention or treatment of colon and breast cancers, type 2 diabetes and cardiovascular diseases.

16. **Lycopene** - Lycopene is well known specifically to help prevent many forms of cancer as well as the prevention and treatments of many illnesses and diseases such as cardiovascular diseases. Lycopene stops LDL cholesterol from being oxidized by free radicals and as such doesn't contribute to the arterial plaque which narrows and hardens the arteries. Infertility research suggests that lycopene may help in the treatment of infertility. Results from tests showed that lycopene can boost sperm concentration in men. Other benefits: it helps prevent diabetes, prevents age-related macular degeneration and cataracts, prevents the aging of the skin and keeps it younger looking, acts as an internal sunscreen and protects your skin from sunburn. Lycopene is also shown to help prevent osteoporosis.

17. **Magnesium** – Among the major and minor minerals needed by the body to achieve maximum health status, magnesium stands out as a stellar performer. Deficiency of this critical mineral is closely associated with mental disorders, depression, vertigo, muscular weakness, nervous conditions, insomnia, cramps, and spasms. A major component of plant-derived chlorophyll, itself a wonderful supplement, magnesium is widely known to affect prevention of osteoporosis, ease symptoms of PMS, is a powerful antioxidant, helps prevent heart disease, lowers blood pressure, helps to prevent diabetes, combats chronic fatigue syndrome and kidney stones, as well as helps to maintain muscle mass.

18. **Melatonin** – A powerful antioxidant, it is neuroprotective, used for treatment of ocular diseases, Parkinson's, post-stroke treatment, hypertension, blood disorders, gastrointestinal tract diseases, cardiovascular diseases, diabetes, rheumatoid arthritis, fibromyalgia, chronic fatigue syndrome, infectious diseases, neurological diseases, sleep disturbances, aging, depression, macular degeneration, glaucoma, protection of the stomach lining (gastric mucosa), irritable bowel syndrome, hypertension and diabetes. Melatonin also helps combat the effects of chemotherapy and radiation, alleviates sleep disorders associated with the circadian rhythm, useful against ulcerative colitis, Crohn's disease, rheumatoid arthritis, cancer treatment (especially that of the prostate), and prevents migraine headaches. Melatonin is naturally produced in the pineal gland yet many natural health advocates are increasingly pointing out its value as a supplement.

19. **Men's Daily Vitamin and Mineral** – When one considers taking daily supplements, I highly recommend avoiding the more commercially marketed types as they are too often made of chemical substances, artificial ingredients, and industrial byproducts. Among the ingredients which must be included in one's daily supplement, and herein I am sharing my own supplements (I'll focus on women's critical nutrients in a later chapter), my all-in-one men's daily supplement includes vitamins A, C, D, E & K, a spectrum of B vitamins including thiamin (B1), riboflavin (B2), niacin (B3), pantothenic acid (B5), pyridoxine (B6) and cyanocobalamin (B12), folic acid, as well as minerals such as calcium, selenium, copper, chromium, natural fluoride, iron, magnesium, manganese and zinc. Depending on the manufacturer, other ingredients may be included as well. My choice includes saw palmetto, spirulina, lycopene, green vegetable powder, and a spectrum of digestive enzymes along with a probiotic.

20. **Milk Thistle** – An extract of the seeds of a common European plant, milk thistle has been exported around the world. It is nontoxic and can be used for extended periods. If you are concerned about stresses on your liver from alcohol, street drugs, medications, abnormal liver function, exposure to solvents or any other toxic exposures, milk thistle should be taken regularly. As powerful as this herb is, it has no known toxic effects.

21. **Modified Citrus Pectin (MCP)** – Another of my favorite detox supplements, MCP is associated with significantly increasing the urinary excretion of heavy metal toxins (hence a need to drink lots of purified water when using this agent) as well as inhibiting tumor growth and metastasis (the spread of cancer to other sites within the body). Unless one has known citrus fruit allergies, there is very little chance that any negative side effects will be experienced. Recommended to be taken on an empty stomach, MCP's cancer-fighting ability is believed to arise from its interaction with a class of specialized proteins called galectin-binding lectins. Galectins are carbohydrate-binding proteins that help the cells clump together more easily, thereby facilitating the growth and spread of certain types of cancer. These are associated with processes involved in cancer, such as adhesion, migration, progression, and metastasis. It is reported that MCP helps fight cancers by binding with galectin-3 to decrease cancer cell aggregation, adhesion, and metastasis.

22. **Parasite Cleanse** – Widely available in various compounds, ParaCleanse™ is another of my favorite seasonal detoxification agents. While we may be alert to the need to periodically cleanse pets of parasites, few people, even pet owners themselves, consider a corresponding need for our own such treatment. Without going into the long list of intestinal and systemic parasites that humans are known to encounter throughout their lives, suffice to say that parasitic infections can range from no symptoms to the most devastating symptoms affecting all the body's organs; the worst of which can lead to death and major disorders. Symptoms of parasitic infection include abdominal pain, constipation or diarrhea, vomiting, systemic infection, joint pain, migraine headaches, malabsorption of nutrients, chronic fatigue, and even parasite-associated risk of developing cancer (liver flukes from seafood, aka cholangiocarcinogenesis). Ingredients common to parasite cleansing compounds include black walnut hull, Graviola bark, wormwood, clove, pumpkin seed, aloe vera, garlic, Diatomatious Earth, Sweet Annie (also known as Artemisia annua or sweet wormwood), and other natural herbs. I commit to a parasite cleanse every 90 days and I also attempt to limit or avoid contact with areas common to indoor pets.

23. **Plant Enzymes** – These enzymes are critically important toward taking the load off the pancreas and other sources of digestive enzymes, thus allowing the body to shift its enzyme-producing capacities more toward the critically important metabolic enzymes, found throughout the whole of the body's cellular, organ and adrenal gland functioning.

24. **Potassium Citrate** – Potassium is one of the 8 major minerals responsible for health and one of the critically-needed minerals and electrolytes that regulate the balance of fluids throughout the body. Potassium citrate, a potassium salt of citric acid, is involved in nerve function, muscle control (including the heart muscle), blood pressure regulation, reducing the risk of kidney stones, reducing the risk of stroke and combating osteoporosis by increasing the bone-beneficial effect of calcium.

25. **Pregnenolone** – This powerful nutraceutical is often paired or linked with DHEA in that it is referred to as the "grand precursor" that is the bases of nearly all steroid hormone production in the body. Naturally-produced hormones that we produce from pregnenolone which are critical to health and function include DHEA, cortisol, testosterone, several estrogens, and the uterus-associated hormone progesterone. Pregnenolone supplementation is useful for combatting fatigue and increasing energy, recovering from traumatic injury, boosting immunity, combatting stress, skin disorders like psoriasis and scleroderma, fibrocystic breast disease (lumpy breasts), endometriosis, menopause symptoms, premenstrual syndrome (PMS), improving cardiovascular function, treating autoimmune disorders such as lupus, sarcoidosis and multiple sclerosis (MS), prostate problems, seizures, stimulating brain function, improving REM sleep, enhancing learning and memory, beneficial mood impact including anxiety and depression, increases levels of other neurosteroids,, decreases cell death, combats inflammation, decrease the rate of multiple degenerative diseases, and "sustains optimal cognitive function in maturing individuals." Make sure your purchase "bioidentical pregnenolone" when shopping for this supplement to assure that you are not obtaining it from animal-based sources. For so many reasons this

has become one of my most valued additions to my arsenal of anti-aging supplements.

26. **Probiotic Acidophilus** – We have a tremendous spectrum of beneficial bacterial flora which inhabits our gut, (estimated to be as high as 100 trillion cells) that are integral to proper digestive function. It is imperative that this gut *microbiome* is as healthy as possible. Also found in other parts of the body, including the mouth and vagina, well-balanced acidophilus is associated with optimal blood pressure and cholesterol (balancing the ratio between HDL and LDL), strengthening immune system function, healthy infant digestion (transferred through breastfeeding), reducing the severity of allergies, aiding in a spectrum of digestive conditions, fighting against the invasion of Candida Albicans (yeast infection), fighting ulcers and staph infections, increasing nutrient absorption, preventing or repairing leaky gut syndrome, and helping to balance the pH of the upper intestinal tract, thus reducing the symptoms of heartburn. As well, health-enhancing acidophilus helps to produce natural antibiotic substances such as acidolin, acidophillin, lactobacillin, lactocin, and others. Published benefits of a healthy gut-bacterial balance are even more extensive. Vegans should be careful to obtain acidophilus from non-dairy sources.

27. **Rhodiola Rosea** – Also known as Arctic Root, this is a most amazing herb under the class of nutriceuticals known as adaptogens, touted for their ability to balance the body's hormonal system. From a massive amount of scientific studies accumulating around the world, especially from Europe and Asia, benefits of Rhodiola include fighting fatigue and depression, increasing physical endurance, treating impotence, preventing altitude sickness, increasing resistance to a spectrum of biological, chemical and physical stressors, and increasing the production of cellular energy (ATP), the loss of which among the elderly is believed to be an underlying culprit behind most degenerative diseases. It is said that, because much of this research on Arctic Root took place in the Soviet Union during the Cold War, that many Americans are very unfamiliar with the extensive research on this herb that could be beneficial to those of us seeking to combat the effects of aging naturally.

28. **Saw Palmetto** – Of undeniable concern among aging men are issues related to prostate health, the overall effects of shifting hormone levels affected by aging, as well as environmental stresses from endocrine disrupting chemicals we constantly encounter. Among the various challenges men face are rising incidences of benign prostatic hypertrophy (BPH), which affects many men from the age of 40, and which can result in moderate-to-severe lower urinary tract symptoms that impact one's quality of life. Another great concern is the rising incidence of prostate cancer among men, especially within the most developed countries. Numerous benefits of the herbal supplement saw palmetto include modulating hormonal effects, preventing hair loss, positive effects of zinc supplementation (zinc is a major component of the herb), combating or preventing inflammatory conditions in the reproductive tract, and it is a powerful agent for strategies to rejuvenate one's hormonal balance. For women as well as men, supplementation with this herb is associated with increased libido. For women, a suggested daily dose of 160 mg is half of that recommended for men, which will range from 160-320 mg daily.

29. **Schizandra Berry** – Native to parts of China, the fruit of *Schizandra Chinensis* has more than 2,000 years of historical record as a powerful agent within both Chinese and Japanese medicine. One of the most widely touted adaptogens, Schizandra is shown beneficial for improving cardiac function and pulmonary diseases (relating to combined cardiac and respiratory function), combating respiratory problems, useful cancer prevention or treatment compound, combating liver disease, has anti-inflammatory properties, as well as useful for decreasing free radical formation.

30. **Selenium** – This critical mineral is regarded by many to be, like magnesium, a super-mineral, with benefits ranging from a powerful immune system booster, to promoting youthfulness, useful for immunodeficiency patients, beating back such hallmarks of aging as vulnerability to acute diseases, as well as protocols for preventing and treating both cancer and heart disease. Selenium is particularly recommended to reduce the risk of prostate and colon cancer. It is also thought to help prevent blood clots, heart attack, and stroke by helping to keep blood platelets from clumping together.

Additionally, along with the antioxidant glutathione, selenium works to bind toxic heavy metals in the body (mercury, lead, and cadmium), thus serving as a chelating agent. It is useful for detoxifying oxidized fats, alcohol, tobacco smoke as well as both legal and street drugs.

31. **Spirulina** – As a "superfood superstar," spirulina is one nutritional source that bridges food and supplementation. Because its taste is not necessarily appealing for most people, taking it in capsulated form, tablets or as an addition to smoothies is advised. It has the greatest concentration of protein of any known food source, much higher than meat products, eggs or dairy. Spirulina is a bacterial organism grown in both fresh and seawater, often referred to as super blue-green algae. This superfood is loaded with not only protein but several B vitamins, copper, iron, magnesium, potassium, and manganese, along with the entire spectrum of micronutrients. Gram for gram, spirulina is considered to be the most nutritious food on the planet providing nutritional benefits to include antioxidant and anti-inflammatory uses, lowering blood triglyceride and LDL levels, preventing or helping to treat oral cancer, reduce blood pressure, prevent hyperglycemia, improve symptoms of nasal allergies, combat anemia and strengthen muscles while improving endurance.

32. **Stinging Nettle Extract** – As we age, our ability to produce hormones associated with reproduction naturally declines. Among men (and to a lesser extent women as well), the decline in free testosterone is associated with male prostate problems, can contribute to muscle wasting, and speeds up aging processes among both sexes. One of the strategies that one can use to prevent this is using Stinging Nettle Extract supplement which not only helps to "prevent the binding of sex hormone-binding globulin to testosterone", which will allow more free testosterone to circulate, but these lignans also nutritionally reinforce the base of amino acids which provide material for the manufacture of hormones.

33. **Trimethylglycine (TMG)** – This powerful substance is manufactured by the body as well as found within various food substances, such as cooked vegetables. With no known adverse effects, TMG benefits include reducing the risk of heart disease and cancer, assisting in the regulation and expression of genetics, helping to remove toxic

metals and chemicals, and assisting in the process of millions of biochemical reactions because it easily donates one or two methyl groups, necessary for complex reactions on the cellular level. TMG is also beneficial in lowering homocysteine levels (associated with inflammation and hardening of the arteries), cardiovascular health, liver detoxification, alleviating depression and mental traumas, reducing risk of diabetes, facilitating DNA expression, as well as aiding in the function of glycine in the formation of collagen, thus promoting healthy formation and functioning of connective tissues such as tendons, ligaments, cartilage, arteries, veins, skin and other such structures. Because of such a variety of uses, supplementation with TMG is highly recommended as an anti-aging strategy.

34. **Vitamin B-12** – Also known as cobalamin and cyanocobalamin, vitamin B-12 supplementation is of concern for vegetarians and vegans, as one of the chief dietary sources for this critical nutrient in the Western diet is meat. While plant food sources such as whole grains can provide enough supply, the persistence of vitamin B-12 deficiency in the elderly, which can range as high as 50 percent, is of concern. Deficiency of this critical vitamin is associated with pernicious anemia, oral inflammation, peripheral neuropathy (numbness or tingling in the extremities), mental disorders such as deterioration, dementia, psychosis and depression, chronic fatigue syndrome, diarrhea, poor appetite and "children's growth failure." Vitamin B-12 is involved in the breakdown of protein, carbohydrates, and fats, the production of red and white blood cells, along with blood platelets. Among the many ways that B-12 supplementation fights aging is that it mediates fatty acid metabolism and serves to reduce blood levels of homocysteine (a risk factor for atherosclerosis and stroke). B-12 is also believed to prevent irreversible neurological damage and improve one's overall blood profile, preventing anemia.

35. **Vitamin C / Ascorbic Acid** – Long known as one of the most important nutrition components of a healthy life, as an anti-aging agent, vitamin C's role is critical. As we combat the devastating effects of free radical damage, resolve inflammatory conditions, balance our blood cholesterol towards the health-promoting HDL, and reduce risk from atherosclerosis, vitamin C's importance as a key nutrient loom ever larger. The long list of benefits associated with

adequate vitamin C levels includes preventing scurvy, treating acute infections (colds, flu), overall boosting the immune system, lowering hypertension, detoxifying lead poisoning, promoting wound healing, treating cancer, combating stroke, for skin elasticity, controlling asthma, and reversing cataracts.

36. **Vitamin E & Tocotrienol Complex** – Vitamin E is a powerful antioxidant which protects cell membranes, preserves enzyme sites, protects DNA from free radical damage, treatment for stroke-induced injuries, various cancers (pancreatic, hepatic, breast, prostate and skin cancer), cholesterol reduction, diabetes treatment, as well as aids in detoxification from radiation exposure. Tocotrienols are an extension of the vitamin E complex.

I am proud to share this list of supplements from within my own personal supply. By no means is this a comprehensive list. Yet I trust that you can see that I take this subject of longevity-associated *hyper nutrition* very seriously. When one considers the number of these super-supplements that are intended to prevent cancer and other chronic diseases, we thus have established great justification for further research and tactical planning.

I do not take all these supplements at one time and don't recommend anyone to do so. I generally will take no more than 6 to 12 supplements at a time and then wait at least 12 hours before taking the same or another set. As well, I do not take supplements every day; I may go weeks without using any at all. My daily diet of Living Superfood is itself one of the best regimens for consistently accessing high-quality nutrients, of a broad spectrum, in the most easily digestible form. Still, my acquired nutritional intelligence, along with a strong intuitive sense, moves me from time to time to bring these supplements forward in order to rebalance, fine-tune and super-energize my body's metabolic functions.

Later in the book, I will focus further on specific nutritional supplements which are complementary to women's and men's distinct needs. Meanwhile, I hope that this peek into my own supplement storehouse has been inspiring and informative to aid you toward your commitment to achieving high-quality life extension

# Chapter 15 – **Why Do Vegans and Vegetarians Live Longer?**

## Comparing Okinawa, Paleo and Raw Vegan Diets for Longevity

One would practically have to have been living in a remote cave to not having encountered the often-heated debate as to which nutrition lifestyle is better for health – that of the vegan/vegetarian or omnivore? This was subject of several of my investigative broadcasts, during which I featured extensive sets of data-based analyses, exposing both sides of the debate. Numerous studies, from a spectrum of reliable institutions, have cited as references. To appear fair and balanced, we put into the record several arguments which counter the supremacy of veganism as the optimal nutritional style. In any case, we must accept that people are free to make their own choices as to whether to eat meat, eggs, seafood, and dairy. As well, we note that the consequences of such choices are far-ranging and substantial. As a rule, I believe that *informed choice* allows for the best choice.

Nutrition consultant, blogger Anthea Frances, responded to an email posing a challenge of comparisons among her own mostly-raw vegan diet, the Okinawa Diet that she had been writing about as one of the best diets for longevity, and the omnivorous eating style referred to as the Paleo diet, which promotes the idea that human ancestors included animal flesh in their diet while avoiding grains. Ms. Frances posted the following response for her Real Raw Nutrition blog [70]:

> From my reading on the topic, there appears to be substantial anthropological research pointing to our frugivorous nature and origins, as well as a number of stories of modern humans who have reversed chronic disease to thrive and live long lives on Fruit-based diets... However, the science for fruit is often completely overwhelmed by sponsored scientific

---

[70] What's the Best Diet for Longevity? Okinawa? Paleo? Raw Vegan?, by Anthea Frances, Feb. 2015, www.RealRawNutrition.com

research and dietary propaganda coming from the agriculture industry and that's why we get confused.

Frances pointed out distinctions between this fruit and vegetable lifestyle and that of dietary proponents for Paleo, one of which claimed that "we were Paleolithic hunters and would have eaten meat as our primary sustenance but were not designed for grains." Another authority claimed that "starch ought to be the basis of our diet." Yet another claimed, "we ate mostly starchy vegetables, with a little fruit and very small amounts of animal flesh and products." This debate certainly can leave people confused, thus likely to opt for the model most closely resembling the one they are already consuming.

So, Frances turned to the investigations of anthropologists and naturalist scientists who based their nutrition research on the anatomical structure of the human body in order to determine the basis of our dietary evolution. What they found was indicative of which foods most closely matched our physiological evolution.

By comparing our teeth, digestive tracts, bipedal physical structure, arms, hands and fingers and our natural inclinations faced with various types of 'food', naturalists have concluded that humankind belongs in the category of the frugivora (that is, primarily fruit eaters, with the addition of plants, nuts and seeds).

The Frenchman, Baron George Cuvier (1769-1832), perhaps the greatest naturalist of the 19th Century, said that humans appear to be formed to nourish themselves chiefly on fruits, the succulent parts of vegetables, and roots based on a study of their anatomical structure.

The shape of their hands, the shortness and moderate strength of their jaws, the equal length of canine and other teeth and the round tubular-like shape of their molars would not permit humans to graze or to devour meat, but rather to pick and gather the harvest of the garden and orchard. [71]

---

[71] Ibid, Anthea Frances

In her article, the author emphasizes that an *idealized* diet is suited to the individual, and should be based upon extensive personal research, with a strong emphasis on balancing protein, fat, and carbohydrates in the form of fruit and starches. She points out that "you have to start listening to your own body and letting it guide you towards the healthiest diet, rather than being tossed around on a turbulent sea of other people's opinions." I certainly do agree with this perspective even though we cannot logically dismiss the sheer physics of our anatomy and how it differs from true omnivores and carnivores.

Which animals live longer, vegetarians or meat eaters?

When we consider longevity in animals, we can compare vegetarians, omnivores and carnivores to see which, on average, live longer. This is not necessarily the easiest of comparisons when one considers that large animals can live so much longer than small ones. Yet, we can get gain more insight into these links between diet and longevity with a few carefully selected examples, focusing on larger species and human-like primates.

- Primates – Comparing the omnivore chimpanzee to the vegetarian gorilla shows that the advantage favors the gorilla, whose anatomical structure is closely related to that of human physiology. Wild gorillas have an average lifespan between 35 and 40 years with some zoo species reaching 50 years and more. The longest-lived gorilla on record is today 59 years of age. Similarly, the average lifespan of a chimpanzee is from 40 to 50 years in the wild while zoo species can live from 50-60 years. It should be noted that diet for all zoo primates, which can include meat-eating for certain species, most often emphasize high amounts of vitamin C and crude fiber for the animals to maintain optimal health. Another indicator that plant-based zoo feeding is preferred is the emphasis on unsaturated fatty acids. Many zoo species of primates are fed protein biscuits, low in saturated fats and of very high fiber content. A zoo primate feeding manual stated that when these protein biscuits are not available in sufficient amounts, "greens and vegetables can be a replacement..." Nowhere did I find any preferred diet for chimps and other large primates that promoted increasing meat consumption for the animals' health. [72]

- Large land species – In an earlier chapter of this book, we looked at average lifespan among various species. The longest living land species were tortoises from Galapagos (172 years) and Aldabra (152 years), both of whom are strictly vegetarian. Their diet consisted of cactus, leaves, grass, berries and sea moss. Captive tortoises similarly had a vegetarian diet, reportedly "similar to that of horses, Asian elephants, and Indian rhinoceroses, all hindgut-fermenting herbivores." [73] Lifespan for large herbivore species can be quite instructive for the purpose of our comparative analysis: African elephants (60-70 years), Asian elephants (48 years), rhinoceros (35-50 years), hippopotamus (40-50), and giraffes (25-28 years). We can then compare those to the average lifespan for carnivores: wild polar bears (20 years), Kodiak bears (25-30 years), crocodiles (70-100 years), tigers (20-26 years), lions (10-14 years), hyenas (12 years), anaconda snakes (10-12 years), and wolves (6-8 years). When comparing the largest herbivore and carnivore species, the average length of lifespan definitely favors herbivores. While the longest living carnivore, the crocodile, could live to be as much as 100 years of age, this pales in comparison to its distant cousin the vegetarian tortoise which can live to be twice as long.

- Bird species – We further compare birds such as wild grey parrots (vegetarian, 80 years), Hyacinth macaws (vegetarian, 50 years), cockatoos (vegetarians, 75 years), albatrosses (fish-eating carnivore, 42 years), various species of vultures (carnivores, 10-30 years), and eagles (carnivores, 20 years). As with large land mammals, the longevity edge goes firmly to vegetarian birds.

## Statistics on vegetarianism and health outcome

It is not difficult these days to access studies comparing the long-term health advantages of various diets. There should be little argument that the (largely-substandard) Standard American Diet can be expected to

---

[72] Nutrition in Primates, from the Merck Veterinary Manual, 2015 revision edition.
[73] Galapagos Tortoise, *Chelonoidis nigra*, Taxonomy & Nomenclature, May 2010, from the library of the San Diego, CA. zoo.

yield a poor outcome with regard to long term health status among its adherents. We should prefer to compare among more conscious eating styles to come to determine if indeed completely eliminating meat, eggs, dairy, fish and animal-based proteins should produce the greatest advantage in disease risk reduction.

We can then consider the next stage of evolving for conscious eaters beyond vegetarian to that of an organic-preferring vegan who avoids animal-based proteins in the diet along with long chain chemical molecules (artificial flavors, excitotoxins, artificial colorings, and chemical preservatives). As well, other food contaminants such as endocrine disrupting chemicals, farm chemicals, pesticide residues, byproducts of GMO farming, and numerous other modern components have been proven to compromise the integrity of our food.

*Business Insider* discussed this issue of nutrition and health in an October 2013 article, "**7 Charts That Could Convince You To Become A Vegetarian**." While the bulk of the article emphasized great benefits to the planetary environment which would follow should the world move further towards the vegetarian lifestyle, one section of the article highlighted a chart on Nutrition and Health which compared the range of micronutrients within a spectrum of common foods:

> The graph below shows the Aggregate Nutrient Density Index for various foods. Dr. Joel Fuhrman created the system on a scale of one to 1,000 by evaluating an extensive range of micronutrients, including vitamins, minerals, phytochemicals, and antioxidant capacities.
>
> The most nutrient-rich foods are all vegetables, like mustard greens which score 100 [SIC – This number for mustards actually reads *1000* on the ANDI Guide]. One cup has 1.6 grams of protein, 1.8 grams of fiber, 65% of your daily Vitamin C, 33% daily Vitamin A, among other nutrients.

The highest-rated animal product on the list, fish, scores only 15; red meat scores only eight. While animal products are high in protein and iron, they lack other vital nutrients.[74]

The *Business Insider* article went on to cite research on the topic from the American Society of Clinical Nutrition which concluded: "current prospective cohort data from adults in North America and Europe raise the possibility that a lifestyle pattern that includes a very low meat intake is associated with greater longevity." Their research also correlated longer lifespan with lifelong exposure to the vegetarian discipline, noting that "long-term vegetarians (17 or more years) live 3.6 years longer than short-term vegetarians."

Such prestigious medical publications as the *Journal of the American Medical Association (JAMA), Internal Medicine,* have similarly featured research which links a vegetarian diet to lower mortality rates. A 2013 article written by Camille Burch for the *Purdue Exponent,* entitled **"Studies show vegetarians live longer,"** began with a quote from Albert Einstein and then went on to point to several longevity advantages enjoyed by vegetarians over their meat-eating study cohorts:

"Nothing will benefit human health and increase the chances for survival of life on Earth as much as the evolution to a vegetarian diet," said Einstein.

Recently, a study published in the Journal of the American Medicine Association Internal Medicine showed an association between a vegetarian diet and lower mortality rates. The results show that, of the people studied, compared to non-vegetarians, vegetarians had a 12 percent lower risk of dying. The study also looked at several other diets that include reduced or no meat consumption. Vegans were found to have a 15 percent lower risk of dying, and people whose meat consumption is limited to seafood had a 19 percent lower risk of death.

---

[74] 7 Charts that Could Convince You to Become A Vegetarian, Christina Sterbenz and Gus Lubin, Business Insider, Oct 2013

The results show a strong enough correlation to entice meat eaters to trade steak for broccoli; although before doing so, people should weigh in variables that may have affected the results, including amount of exercise. [75]

This article, as well as the study cited, did note that *pesco vegetarians*, whose only meat consumption was from seafood, enjoyed an even greater reduction in risk of death during the study period, a 19% lowered risk compared to the 15% risk reduction enjoyed by vegetarians.

## The myth of vegan centenarians?

Elsewhere in this book, we examined four longevity-associated populations within regions around the world that were highlighted in Dan Buettner's book *The Blue Zones*. His research began with a particularly in-depth analysis of the elderly in Okinawa, Japan, whose population boasts the highest average life expectancy of any region in the world. Advocates of the omnivorous diet have been quick to point out that Okinawan centenarians do consume meat and seafood, thus making a presumptive conclusion that vegetarianism is not necessarily superior to being an omnivore when in pursuit of long life expectancy. The following analysis presents an alternative assessment of the Okinawa diet and points to the relatively small amounts of meat and seafood that have been consumed during the lifetime of the island's noteworthy centenarians.

What follows is from a transcript to the documentary film produced by Michael Greger, M.D., *The Okinawa Diet: Living to 100*.

The traditional diet in Okinawa is based on vegetables, beans, and other plants. I'm used to seeing the Okinawan diet represented like this—the base being vegetables, beans, and grains, but a substantial contribution from fish and other meat. But a more accurate representation would be this, if you look at their actual dietary intake. We know what they were eating from the U.S. National Archives, because the U.S. military ran Okinawa until it was given back to Japan in

[75] Does a vegetarian diet really increase longevity? by CAMILLE BURCH The Exponent, Jun 12, 2013, www.PurdueExponent.org

1972. And if you look at the traditional diets of more than 2,000 Okinawans, this is how it breaks down.

Less than 1% of their diet was fish; less than 1% of their diet was meat, and same with dairy and eggs, so it was more than 96% plant-based, and more than 90% whole food plant based—very few processed foods either. And, not just whole food plant-based, but most of their diet was vegetables, and one vegetable in particular—sweet potatoes. The Okinawan diet was centered around purple and orange sweet potatoes—how delicious is that? Could have been bitter gourd, or soursop—but no, sweet potatoes, yum.

So, 90 plus percent whole food plant-based makes it a highly anti-inflammatory diet, makes it a high antioxidant diet. If you measure the level of oxidized fat within their system, there is compelling evidence of less free radical damage. Maybe they just genetically have better antioxidant enzymes or something? No, their antioxidant enzyme activity is the same; it's all the extra antioxidants that they're getting from their diet that may be making the difference—most of their diet is vegetables! [76]

## Reduce meat consumption, live longer

It should be very easy to determine from studies published across a broad array of medical science journals that we can significantly reduce the incidence of life-threatening chronic diseases by lowering the percentage of calories we consume daily from meat, eggs and dairy products. Macro studies conducted by researchers give us access to a larger set of studies and, subsequently, a wide array of study subjects and lifestyle conditions.

*Time Magazine*, in an article by Alexandra Sifferlin in 2014, cited one such macro study published in the journal *JAMA Internal Medicine*, entitled "**7 Reasons Vegetarians Live Longer**." Sifferlin cited seven clinical studies, along with 32 other studies spanning the years 1900 to

[76] Transcript: The Okinawa Diet: Living to 100, by Michael Greger, M.D., from www.NutritionFacts.org, Oct 2015

2013. Among this broad set of studies their findings clearly pointed to the reasons that vegetarians tend to outlive "meat-lovers" [77]:

1. Vegetarians have lower blood pressure on average, and they found that "a vegetarian diet can be used to lower blood pressure when intervention was necessary."

2. In a study of over 70,000 people, vegetarians were shown to have a 12% lower risk of death over non-vegetarians and a lower risk for chronic diseases overall.

3. Vegetarians scored better on mood tests than those who ate omnivore or fish-only diets.

4. Citing a study of 44,000 people, vegetarians were 32% less likely to suffer from cardiovascular disease, the number one cause of death each year in the U.S.

5. Researchers at California's Loma Linda University examined differing versions of the vegetarian diet and found significantly lowered risk for cancers; "specifically cancers most common among women, like breast cancer." It is widely known that high fiber diets common to vegetarianism lower the risk of certain cancers such as colon and stomach cancer.

6. Vegetarians are at a lower risk of developing diabetes. While not noted in the Time Magazine article, extensive research firmly shows that strict vegan diet, combined with stress reduction, exercise, and supplementation, has a remarkable track record in actually reversing type-2 diabetes in as little as 21 to 30 days.

7. Vegetarians are less likely to be obese or overweight, in addition to lower plasma levels of LDL cholesterol and reduced body mass index (BMI). Converting to a vegetarian diet has long been associated with maintaining a healthy weight profile over time.

This particular article, which mirrors so many others that compare the health benefits of vegetarian, vegan and meat-eating lifestyles, goes on to point out that not all vegetarians are healthy (a fact with which this

[77] 7 Reasons Vegetarians Live Longer, by Alexandra Sifferlin, Feb 24, 2014, Time Magazine online

author firmly agrees) and that not all meat eaters function in poor health. What we can say with confidence is that as one is looking for additional tools or lifestyle habits to adopt toward the aim of longevity, disease avoidance and maintenance of youthful vitality, becoming a vegetarian or vegan will definitely present a significant advantage.

## Eating red meat is linked to cancer and inflammation

********** BREAKING NEWS ********** You've probably seen this disruptive alert flash across your television screen and, predictably, your attention is instantly focused on the immediate story to follow – this could be some threat that directly affects your safety, a nearby emergency or some other issue of urgent concern. Yet we don't get these types of alerts when there is a new research study finding that might potentially impact the lives of thousands of people. As an example, have any of us ever received an emergency alert warning that *24,000 Americans will die* this year of antibiotic-resistant bacteria encountered in the meat and dairy supply as well as acquired in hospitalized settings?

One such alert that should have gained urgent attention was issued from the University of California, San Diego School of Medicine in late December 2014; it quickly caught my attention. During my morning news scan, I came across this alarming press release detailing a health research study that utilized specially-developed laboratory mice that, just like humans, were genetically engineered to be incapable of processing a specialized *sugar-like molecule, Neu5Gc*, which was found in red meat (e.g., pork, beef, bison and lamb). [78] The UCSD findings showed that human's inability to process Neu5Gc increased rates of chronic inflammation by as much as 500%. They further concluded that this inflammatory condition was a known factor for increasing tumor formation, with the Neu5Gc protein being found encapsulated within the tumors. This failure to process this substance was not found within any other meat-eating species. To quote from that press release:

---

[78] Sugar Molecule Links Red Meat Consumption and Elevated Cancer Risk in Mice, December 23, 2014, by Heather Buschman, PhD, UC San Diego Health, from the campus website

In a study published in the Dec. 29 online early edition of the *Proceedings of the National Academy of Sciences*, the scientists found that feeding Neu5Gc to mice engineered to be deficient in the sugar (like humans) significantly promoted spontaneous cancers. The study did not involve exposure to carcinogens or artificially inducing cancers, further implicating Neu5Gc as a key link between red meat consumption and cancer.

"Until now, all of our evidence linking Neu5Gc to cancer was circumstantial or indirectly predicted from somewhat artificial experimental setups," said principal investigator Ajit Varki, MD, Distinguished Professor of Medicine and Cellular and Molecular Medicine and member of the UC San Diego Moores Cancer Center. "This is the first time we have directly shown that mimicking the exact situation in humans — feeding non-human Neu5Gc and inducing anti-Neu5Gc antibodies — increases spontaneous cancers in mice."

Of various alarming conclusions from this study, researchers: 1) "hypothesized that eating red meat could lead to inflammation if the body's immune system is constantly generating antibodies against consumed animal Neu5Gc, a foreign molecule." 2) "the scientists found that feeding Neu5Gc to mice engineered to be deficient in the sugar (like humans) significantly promoted spontaneous cancers." and 3) "this work may also help explain potential connections of red meat consumption to other diseases exacerbated by chronic inflammation, such as atherosclerosis and type 2 diabetes."

\*\*\*\*\*\*\*\*\*\* END OF EMERGENCY ALERT \*\*\*\*\*\*\*\*\*\*

## Dairy, lactose intolerance and chronic inflammation

For most of my life now I, like many others, have completely avoided all dairy products: milk, cheese, cream, butter, ice cream as well as processed foods manufactured with the milk proteins lactose and casein. Decades ago I was alerted to the book by Frank A. Oski, M.D., ***DON'T DRINK YOUR MILK!: New Frightening Medical Facts about the World's Most Overrated Nutrient***. While my own awakening to the dangerous and deadly impact of milk consumption had earlier become established, reading from Oski's book took me over the top. As Director, Department of Pediatrics, Johns Hopkins University School of Medicine and Physician-in-Chief of the Johns Hopkins Children's Center, Frank Oski was most certainly qualified to be taken seriously in the field of health research.

As the subtitle to the book indicates, this work is a *serious* warning to those who continue to drink milk beyond the age of weaning off of "the world's most over-rated nutrient." In the first chapter, Oski shares many of the hundreds of dire findings exposing the dangerous impact of cow's milk and dairy products on our health:

> The fact is: the drinking of cow milk has been linked to iron-deficiency anemia in infants and children; it has been named as the cause of cramps and diarrhea in much of the world's population, and the cause of multiple forms of allergy as well; and the possibility has been raised that it may play a central role in the origins of atherosclerosis and heart attacks. [79]

I have increasingly pointed to the *absurdity* of the public's dairy-consumption habits within this nation. One question I put forward in my documentary film *Chewicide, the Movie* is, "Can you name one species other than humans which feeds the milk of another species to its children?" On this topic, Oski writes:

> Most lay persons are not aware that the milk of mammalian species varies considerably in its composition. For example, the milk of goats, elephants, cows, camels, yaks, wolves, and walruses show marked differences, one from the other, in their content of fats, protein, sugar, and minerals. Each was designed to provide optimum nutrition to the young of the respective species. Each is different from human milk. [80]

The book also highlights the preponderance of lactose intolerance among various populations of the world, some of which, such as East Asians and Africans, are nearly completely lactose intolerant after the age of 36 months. Oski points out:

---

[79] Don't Drink Your Milk, by Frank A. Oski, M.D., Pg 3
[80] Ibid, Pgs 3-4

In many other parts of the world, most particularly in East Asia, Africa, and South America, people regard cow milk as unfit for consumption by adult human beings. If we are to judge by general mammalian standards their tastes are not peculiar; Americans' and Europeans' tastes are. Despite our notions, it is not the Chinese and Africans who differ most markedly from the norms of nature.

Even prestigious medical science publications have implicated milk consumption in the formation of immune challenge, disease, and disorder, along with associated morbidity and mortality in humans. The *British Medical Journal* published a widely-referenced study in October 2014, entitled "**Milk intake and risk of mortality and fractures in women and men: cohort studies**". Within the extensive published account of their studies, they pointed out that the impact of a sugar-like molecule *D-galactose* had demonstrated negative health impact on those exposed to the substance which was common in dairy products:

A high intake of milk might, however, have undesirable effects, because milk is the main dietary source of D-galactose. Experimental evidence in several animal species indicates that chronic exposure to D-galactose is deleterious to health and the addition of D-galactose by injections or in the diet is an established animal model of aging. Even a low dose of D-galactose induces changes that resemble natural aging in animals, including shortened life span caused by oxidative stress damage, chronic inflammation, neurodegeneration, decreased immune response, and gene transcriptional changes... Based on a concentration of lactose in cow's milk of approximately 5%, one glass of milk comprises about 5 g of D-galactose. The increase of oxidative stress with aging and chronic low-grade inflammation is not only a pathogenetic mechanism of cardiovascular disease and cancer in humans but also a mechanism of age-related bone loss and sarcopenia. The high amount of lactose and therefore D-galactose in milk with theoretical influences on processes such as oxidative stress and inflammation makes the recommendations to increase milk intake for prevention of fractures a conceivable contradiction. [81]

You saw it with your own eyes; the study did say about milk "**Even a low dose of D-galactose induces changes that resemble natural aging in animals, including shortened life span...**" – Now you know why I don't do dairy at all.

Two other key citations in the BMJ article add new elements to the massive body of research exposing the negative health impacts of dairy consumption in humans, and were thus noted in the study's conclusion:

- "A high milk intake in both sexes is associated with higher mortality and fracture rates and with higher levels of oxidative stress and inflammatory biomarkers";

- "Such a pattern was not observed with a high-intake of fermented milk products" – This latter finding would indicate that the normal human gut flora is not naturally conducive to the digestion of milk proteins after weaning, thus cultured dairy products must use exogenous bacteria to break these proteins down into digestible amino acids for human digestion.

The BMJ article stated their findings somewhat conclusively in challenging the highly-touted protective effects of dairy consumption toward the prevention of osteoporosis: "Our results may question the validity of recommendations to consume high amounts of milk to prevent fragility fractures."

## Go vegetarian and save the planet from catastrophe

Many people have committed to the vegan and vegetarian lifestyle because of moral consciousness over the treatment of animals as well as the destructive impact that raising animals for human food has on the sustainability of the nation's environment. My second book in this series, *Living Superfood Research: Don't Get Sick, Stay Off Drugs and Live a Long Time*, contained an extensive chapter called "Grave

---

[81] Milk intake and risk of mortality and fractures in women and men: cohort studies, from the British Medical Journal 2014; 349 doi, October 2014

Dangers from Eating Meat," which pointed out environmental challenges presented by America's obsession with meat:

1. "It is reported that some 29 million pounds of antibiotics were used in 2009 in U.S. meat production alone";

2. "Meat, dairy and eggs introduce dangerous germs into our homes";

3. "Americans consume more meat per capita than any other nation."

With so many food animals being raised industrially in *concentrated animal feedlot operations (CAFOs)*, it should be no surprise that this presents an increasingly greater risk to the sustainability of our natural environment.

One can gather facts on this topic from a vast spectrum of sources. A frequently referenced source is the activist organization *People for the Ethical Treatment of Animals (PETA)*. Their mission goes directly to the heart of this question of the depth of the damage that this nation's high levels of meat production and consumption, presents to the planet's sustainable resources. The following facts are excerpted directly from the PETA.org website:

- Cows must consume 16 pounds of vegetation in order to convert them into 1 pound of flesh. Raising animals for food consumes more than half of all water used in the U.S. It takes 2,500 gallons of water to produce a pound of meat but only 25 gallons to produce a pound of wheat.

- Producing just one hamburger uses enough fossil fuel to drive a small car 20 miles. Of all raw materials and fossil fuels used in the U.S., more than one-third is devoted to raising animals for food.

- A typical pig factory generates the same amount of raw waste as a city of 12,000 people. According to the Environmental Protection Agency, raising animals for food is the number-one source of water pollution.

- Of all agricultural land in the U.S., 87 percent is used to raise animals for food. That's 45 percent of the total land mass in the U.S. About

260 million acres of U.S. forest have been cleared to create cropland to produce feed for animals raised for food. Meat industries are directly responsible for 85 percent of all soil erosion in the U.S.

- More than 80 percent of the corn we grow, and more than 95 percent of the oats are fed to livestock. The world's cattle alone consume a quantity of food equal to the caloric needs of 8.7 billion people—more than the entire human population on Earth. According to the Worldwatch Institute, "Roughly 2 of every 5 tons of grain produced in the world is fed to livestock, poultry, or fish; decreasing consumption of these products, especially of beef, could free up massive quantities of grain and reduce pressure on land." [82]

Considering these and other facts presented within this chapter on the numerous longevity benefits of the vegetarian and vegan lifestyles, one should readily conclude that moving away from eating high amounts of meat, eggs, dairy and seafood can have immediate and long term positive impact on both individual health and environmental sustainability for the benefit of all species.

I do my best to avoid coming off as overly aggressive when advocating for vegetarianism; trying not to come off as what has been referred to as a "vegan Nazi." I find it more productive to *not* beat people over the head, attempting to cajole them into doing something that they are psychologically unprepared to do.

Others, especially food advertisers, have found their greatest successes in deploying techniques to manipulate our emotions toward commercial exploitation. I prefer to continue to collect, analyze and disseminate the facts, trusting that most people can make reasonably sound judgments for their own sake and on their family's behalf.

After rational consideration of these facts, most people should easily agree that the preservation of life, achieving longevity and disease resistance, raising healthy children, protecting our environment and investing our collective resources in preventative healthcare are all good and smart for our nation and our world.

---

[82] How does eating meat harm the environment? / People for the Ethical Treatment of Animals, from PETA.org

With greater cooperation, we are going to do better at outreach, education, and presentation of relevant information to people who are certainly capable of comprehending what is in their best self-interest. Predictably, everybody's not going to understand our lessons to the point of making swift changes in their lifestyle behaviors. Still, we must persist with advocating for truth. We *will* do this for our own preservation of mind, body, and spirit – for a child, friend or loved one – for the family, community or a whole nation – for this generation, the future and for the planet. We will do this because these circles are all so absolutely precious that we must fight unceasingly to protect the sanctity of life. For many of us, this is a sacred mission.

# Chapter 16 – **The Role of Enzymes in Health and Longevity**

*"If humans take in more exogenous (outside) digestive enzymes, as nature ordained, the enzyme potential will not have to waste so much of its heritage digesting food. It can distribute more of this precious commodity to the metabolic enzymes, where it rightfully belongs. This rightful distribution of enzyme energy will not only act to maintain health and prevent disease, but is expected to help cure established disease..."* – Dr. Edward Howell [83]

Our focal point for research in this chapter is largely taken from the book **CONSCIOUS EATING** by Dr. Gabriel Cousens. For most of us, though outside of the spectrum of our conscious attention, enzymes are among the core keys to life and longevity. There are different classes of enzymes that facilitate life processes and those to be found within our food are vital to our well-being. As well, the manners by which food is produced, processed, prepared and consumed greatly affect the integrity of the enzymatic activity that takes place. It is my wholehearted desire that as many of us as possible learn how this spectrum of enzyme activity is connected to literally every fragment of our biology; vital to energy production, disease avoidance and to the expression of our genetic potential.

From the chapter entitled "Enzymes: A Secret of Health and Longevity," we have a wealth of insights from Dr. Cousens and the numerous scientists that he cites on this topic. [84] Setting up the chapter's critical focus on the role of enzymes in all life processes, he offers up quotes

---

[83] Real Food Quote Monday – "Enzyme Nutrition" by Dr. Edward Howell, cited in an article by Wardee Harmon, Sept 2009, from the website of Traditional Cooking School of GNOWFGLINS

[84] Conscious Eating, by Dr. Gabriel Cousens, North Atlantic Books, 1992 / 2000, Pg 519

from several scientists involved in nutrition, microbiological and chemistry research:

- "...enzymes are both chemical protein complexes and bioenergy reservoirs." – Dr. Gabriel Cousens citing the research of Dr. Edward Howell

- Enzymes are "embarrassing because they can do at body temperatures and in simple solution what we organic chemists can do only with corrosive agents and at high temperatures and with laborious processes." – Dr. Robert G. Denkewalter

- "Life is something which has been built up about the enzymes; it is corollary of enzyme activity." – Dr. Leonard Thompson Troland

- "...enzyme preservation is the secret to health." – Ann Wigmore

As well, from another source, the online site of the Traditional Cooking School of GNOWFGLINS, we share this very important revelation, also from Dr. Edward Howell:

> "To get enzymes from food, one must eat raw food. All life, whether plant or animal, requires the presence of enzymes to keep it going."

I have, for over six years now, been primarily on a raw food diet; most likely no more than 3-7 percent of my nutrition being obtained from cooked food during any given month. One of the primary influences for me toward making this dietary transformation was being exposed to nutritional research and healing protocols developed by Dr. Gabriel Cousens. My first exposure to his work was purchasing and viewing the documentary film, *Simply Raw: Reversing Diabetes in 30 Days*. In the film, he and his colleagues treated 6 Americans from diverse backgrounds at a remote healing resort in Arizona. Each subject had been diagnosed as diabetic: four were diagnosed as type-2 diabetes (adult onset) and the other two as type-1 (congenital). The experiment took place at Cousens' Tree of Life Resort in Patagonia, where the six patients were isolated for 30 days (one subject dropped out before the treatment study was completed). Of the five who completed the 30-day experiment, four of them completely reversed their diagnosis of diabetes, including one of the two type-1 diagnosed patients. The second type-1 patient, an alcoholic, had been secretly cheating during the test period yet was still able to cut his daily insulin shot dosage level by over 90%.

That documentary, *Simply Raw*, powerfully impacted my life and I have viewed it along with various groups more than a half-dozen times. After converting to this nutritional style at the Spring Equinox of 2010, I have since collected others of Dr. Cousens' books. I have since built a fairly large collection of books on the raw and superfood culinary arts, as well as added numerous other similar books and films to my library.

Over the course of these six years and more, I've built up a huge digital and print storehouse of thousands of documents covering these areas of advanced nutrition. As well, I've become a widely recognized and authoritative voice around the world presenting the advantages of the raw vegan lifestyle for healing and disease prevention. I even produced my own film on nutrition and disease prevention, *CHEWICIDE, THE MOVIE*. What a wonderful sojourn was set off at this juncture in life.

I have witnessed up close numerous healing miracles which have followed the commitment to raw, vegan, organic superfood nutrition. I've seen this happen in my own life, with loved ones, and among the many dozens of clients that I have assisted as a nutrition consultant. Living Superfood literally changed my life.

I experienced my own healing miracle after having been blindsided by a drunken speeding driver, veered into the curbside parking lane just as I was opening the rear door of my soon-to-be-destroyed minivan. Partly due to my miraculous recovery from that experience, I have since felt obligated to share this miracle with all who would accept it. Yet, getting more people to accept this miraculous gift can often be quite a challenge. This so reminds me of these words, which have been attributed to our great and venerated ancestor Harriet Tubman, – *"I freed thousands of slaves. I could have freed thousands more, if they had known they were slaves."* While there is a dispute as to whether she actually stated these words, for our purpose the idea expressed perfectly suits our mission.

## Three categories of enzymes and their functions

Dr. Cousens points out that there are three categories of enzymes that function within the body; 1) "**metabolic enzymes**, which activate all our systemic functions; 2) **digestive enzymes**, for the processing of food; and a relatively newly conceived category called 3) **food enzymes**." I might provide a quick summary of the relationship between these three classes of enzymes and the question of just *why* the living food lifestyle is preferred. Research confirms that conscious preservation of the integrity of food-borne enzymes allows the body to absorb plant nutrition without having to produce additional reserves of digestive enzymes, thus one enjoys the preservation of the energy that would have been required to fill in this gap. This energy is then available to be directed towards the production of important metabolic enzymes that are needed for a vast spectrum of bodily functions.

Writing on the complexity of enzymatic activity within the body, Dr. Cousens states:

> There are an estimated 50,000 enzymes in the human organism. Approximately 2700-3000 enzymes and their functions have been identified. Each organ has its own set of enzymes. Of the 50,000-plus enzymes, about 24 of them are digestive enzymes. The three main types of digestive enzymes are proteases, which digest proteins; amylases, which digest carbohydrates; and lipases, which digest fats.

He next goes on to point out something very important to our understanding about the need to preserve naturally-occurring enzymes that are part of the plant world, from which we would ideally be taking our nutrition:

> Mother Nature works in conjunction with us by adding what we call from our human-centered point of view "food enzymes" to each living element of nature. These food enzymes have the exact ratio of proteases, amylases, and

lipases required to begin the digestion of the food for the body. [85]

One of the central themes in all my writings on the subject of Living Superfood is that preserving the natural integrity of our nutrition, especially with regard to the preservation of active food enzymes, is one of the principal ways that we actively influence and optimize nutrition outcome. Our stated goal herein is healthy longevity. Thus, the acquisition of lifestyle techniques that preserve food enzyme functionality is a powerful addition to our high-quality life extension tools set.

In a subchapter entitled "The Role of Food Enzymes in Digestion", Dr. Cousens explains in a detailed and information-packed introductory paragraph, several key points that are critical for our comprehension of the importance of both plant and digestive enzymes in our diet:

- There are two distinct sections of the stomach where digestion proceeds;

- The upper stomach retains food for 30-60 minutes and here the breakdown of food relies nearly completely on the "living" enzymes from our food with the contribution of amylase enzyme secreted within our saliva. This is why it is so absolutely important for us to properly chew our food (32 to 48 times before we swallow) in order to insert as much saliva-carried amylase into what we are eating; as well, proper chewing is the means to break the cell walls of the food we consume, facilitating the release of natural enzymes within these plant-based foods.

- The second part of the stomach, called the pyloric stomach, is where hydrochloric acid and pepsin are added to the mix and where the bulk of digestion is carried out. As we know from our larger body of studies, protein digestion carries on throughout the intestinal tract, aided later on by a healthy microbiome of some 100 trillion friendly bacteria that inhabit the gut and work to break down denser proteins through digestive fermentation.

---

[85] Ibid, Conscious Eating Pg 520

One of the more valuable lessons I've learned throughout my lifetime of nutrition studies is the differentiation of digestion when comparing herbivores (plant-eating species) to omnivores (eating both plant foods and flesh) or carnivores (flesh-eating species). Illustrative of the impact of this contrast is the story of the *Pottenger Cats Studies*, which Dr. Cousens cites in this chapter. I originally found this case study so compelling that I sought out much more information about this and other nutrition studies carried out by Francis Pottenger, M.D. Gabriel Cousens wrote:

> Similar animal research was done over a ten-year period by Francis Pottenger, M.D., using 900 cats. He gave half of the cats raw milk and raw meat and the other half pasteurized milk and cooked meat. In the first generation, the cats on the cooked food developed a pattern of degenerative disease similar to what we see in humans. In the second and third generations of cooked-food-eating cats, he observed the onset of congenital bone deformities, hyperactivity, and sterility. The cats became so dysfunctional that plants would not even grow on their manure. The conclusion he made was that some critical, heat-sensitive factor was missing from the cooked food. The main factors known to be completely destroyed by heat are enzymes. [86]

One of the key lessons we derive from this new understanding of the importance of preserving natural plant enzymes in our food is that eating cooked food puts additional stresses on the body's digestive system. This stress is especially difficult on the pancreas as well as the immune system. Dr. Cousens' explains this further:

> The result of this [idealized] digestion in the food enzyme stomach is that the pancreas is not forced to work so hard to secrete so many enzymes. This conserves the body's enzymes for use toward nondigestive, metabolic purposes such as detoxification, repair, and the health and proper functioning of the endocrine glands and other vital organs. Because eating raw foods liberates enzymes for use in other

---

[86] Ibid, Pgs 522-523

parts of the body, the importance of making a high percentage of our diet biogenic and bioactive is obvious.

Evidence compiled by Dr. Howell strongly suggests that eating foods devoid of enzymes as a result of cooking, food irradiation, and microwaving causes an enlargement of the pancreas and also stresses associated endocrine glands, such as the adrenals, pituitary, ovaries, and testes... The most obvious conclusion is that the pancreas becomes hypertrophied, or enlarged, because it is forced to keep up a high digestive enzyme output. [87]

Another of our key takeaways from Dr. Cousens' research is covered within the subchapter "Not Overeating: The Secret to Health, Longevity, and Enzyme Preservation." Here he develops how *caloric restriction* as a longevity strategy is combined with our working knowledge about enzymes, prevention, and recovery from illness. I will admit that this present task of reviewing and excerpting from this book, *Conscious Eating*, is made more difficult because every paragraph contains several absolutely critical points that I want to convey to you, the readers. Yet, the book is over 800 pages in length – you can imagine the amount of highlighting that I've done reviewing this book!

Therefore I will share just a small set of key ideas, from just a few sections of just this one chapter. I hope that you will be inspired to get this or others of Dr. Gabriel Cousens' informative books.

- Dr. Cousens goes on to cite the research "of a Swiss physician, Paul Kouchakoff. In 1930, he showed that the eating of cooked foods caused leukocytosis, which is an increase in white blood cells. This even occurred when water was heated above 191° F. There are two hypotheses to explain this. One is that the white blood cells, which have a similar lipase, protease, and amylase ratio as the pancreas, are actually taking enzymes to the pancreas to boost its supply. The second explanation is that when food is cooked and water boiled, the body recognizes it as foreign and has an immune response to it...the repeated leukocytosis with every meal certainly puts a strain on the immune system. Kouchakoff also found that when subjects started a

---

[87] Ibid, pg 525

meal with raw foods which equaled more than half of the meal, they were able to have some cooked foods and not produce a leukocytosis." (Pgs 525-526)

- "EATING RAW FOODS IS THE NUMBER-ONE ACTIVITY which preserves enzymes and maximizes health. It is the diet of choice of all the rest of Mother Nature's children that dwell on this planet. Animals that live in the wild do not suffer from chronic degenerative diseases as do humans and domesticated animals. It is a striking fact that all other species, without exception, eat their foods raw, whereas the overwhelming majority of humans do not. When animals are fed cooked foods, they to begin to suffer chronic degenerative diseases. ¶ The foods with the highest amount of live enzymes are biogenic, predigested, and fermented foods. Seeds that have the highest enzyme content are those with a ¼ inch sprout." (Pg 528)

- "NOT OVEREATING RAW FOODS is itself another way to conserve enzymes. It is different from an obsessive undereating, which can result in a physical and mental deprivation syndrome. Not overeating is what I call the art of conscious eating. It is learning to take just the right amount of food and drink to support our individual needs on every level of our spiritual and worldly functioning. Researchers have shown that not overeating increases longevity...overeating of even healthy foods was one of the main causes of ill health... ¶ On a 5000-year-old Egyptian pyramid, an inscription of this wisdom was found: 'Man lives on one quarter of what he eats, on the other three quarters, his doctor lives.'" (Pgs 531-532)

- "Live plant digestive enzymes may be the best source of enzyme supplementation. They seem to be active at a much fuller pH range than animal enzymes. These plant enzymes show some activity in the stomach, especially the enzyme stomach, and become immediately active in the small intestine. One study, reported in the Journal of Clinical Nutrition, found that 70% of plant amylase is active in the small intestine after being ingested orally. Because of these facts, I recommend that people consider using plant digestive enzymes for their digestive supplementation." (Pg 533)

- "Enzymes contain the power of the life force itself. Eating a live-food diet helps to maintain the quality and quantity of our enzyme pool and therefore maintain our health and longevity. Enzymes are not simply catalysts that make digestion and all metabolic processes work; they are living proteins that direct the life force into our basic biochemical and metabolic processes. They even help repair our DNA and RNA. Enzymes help transform and store energy, make active hormones, participate in their own production cycle, dissolve fibrin and thus prevent clotting, and have anti-inflammatory effects... The research suggests they also balance and enhance the immune system; help to heal cancer, multiple sclerosis, rheumatoid diseases, and arthritis; minimize the effect of athletic injuries; decrease injury recovery time; and aid with digestion." (Pg 535)

In appreciation of all this and more, I can most certainly testify that Dr. Cousens has researched these topics thoroughly and has provided us with a solid foundation of practical research upon which we can build truly life-transforming habits and behaviors. Who among us will benefit most from taking this live-food, plant-enzyme-rich dietary instruction to heart? He states clearly, "Anyone eating cooked, microwaved, or irradiated food should take food enzyme supplements to compensate for the lost and destroyed naturally occurring food enzymes that were previously in the food." He adds, "During acute and chronic illnesses, there is often an enzyme depletion that can be alleviated by enzyme supplementation."

Let us now have Dr. Cousens issue the last word to those contemplating how living foods, with their living enzymes, along with plant enzyme supplementation, can all contribute not only to life extension, but relieve much of the disease burden that impacts the quality of life for too many during their senior years:

"I have found that people with digestive disturbances, endocrine gland imbalances, blood sugar imbalances, diabetes, obesity, cholesterol excesses, stress-related problems, and arthritic inflammations all seem to benefit from enzyme supplementation." – Dr. Gabriel Cousens, *Conscious Eating*, (Pg 535)

# Chapter 17 –A Review of OXYGEN by Nick Lane

> *"From the dawn of recorded history, its tale of friendship and heroism resonates with the eternal concerns of mankind: bereavement, aging, death, the dream of immortality. These themes recur throughout history, and not just in a vague sense – we cling to the idea that everlasting youth is attainable through the possession of some kind of magical artifact, be it a plant, the nectar of the gods, the Holy Grail, the grated horn of a unicorn, the Elixir of Life, the philosopher's stone, or growth hormones."*
>
> - Nick Lane [88]

## Sex and the Evolution of Aging

In this chapter, we review the book **OXYGEN: The Molecule that Made the World**, by Nick Lane.  For most of us, this author provides a set of radical new perspectives regarding the evolution of life on Earth, biological, molecular and genetic processes, along with a spectrum of *seemingly* unrelated biological mechanisms and their links to longevity. His work details how complex life-cycles of cells have evolved within our species and how so many of our beliefs toward aging have been poorly conceived.  One of the key questions we must consider as we quest for longevity, "Is death a necessary function for genetic survival?"

The history of medical science research in the pursuit of anti-aging and longevity is often filled with theories and practices which today seem ridiculous and barbaric.  Let's peek at 19th-century research into longevity which even went so far as implanting animal testicular organs into humans.  Nick Lane introduces us to this often-sordid history:

---

[88] OXYGEN: The Molecule that Made the World, by Nick Lane, from the chapter Sex and the Art of Bodily Maintenance, Pgs 212-213

Other theories linked aging to men with diminishing testicular secretions. In 1889, Charles Edouard Brown-Sequard, a prominent French physiologist, announced to the Societé de Biologie in Paris that he had rejuvenated his mind and body by injecting himself with a liquid extracted from the testicles of dogs and guinea-pigs. Apparently the injections not only increased his physical strength and intellectual energy, but also relieved his constipation and lengthened the arc of his urine. Later, a number of surgeons tried implanting whole or sliced testicles into the scrotums of recipients. Leo I. Stanley was resident physician in San Quentin prison in California. He began transplanting testicles (removed from recently executed prisoners) into inmates in 1918. Some of the recipients reported full recovery of their sexual potency. By 1920, the scarcity of human gonads induced Stanly to substitute ram, goat, deer and boar testes, which he said worked equally well. He went on to perform hundreds of operations, treating patients with ailments as diverse as senility, asthma, epilepsy, tuberculosis, diabetes and gangrene. [89]

Rick Lane goes on to explain how this madness carried on for decades within the Western medical field with cross-species transplants, organ harvesting, injections with glandular secretions and more. We can still see remnants of such practices carrying on today – the use of DNA containing tissues from 11 different species, including cells from the dissected lungs of aborted fetuses (*human diploid cells*), being the substrate (culture medium) for vaccine production is itself an extension of something that 100 years after the fact will likely look similarly ridiculous.

Lane goes on to bridge this history, which included such characters as "the notorious quack, 'Doctor' John R. Brinkley, another transplant fanatic who made a million-dollar fortune, with the more modern anti-aging efforts of a spectrum of investigators and practitioners.

---

[89] Ibid, Pgs 213-214

Even today, aging is rarely considered a proper field of study within the discipline of medicine – it is still contaminated by the legacy of quacks like Brinkley. In most countries, medical school curricula devote no classes to aging. Yet while turning a blind eye to the study of aging, medicine has accumulated a tremendous wealth of information on the infirmities of old age. This mass of information is all part of gerontology, even though most specialists do not think of themselves as gerontologists, they are cardiologists, neurologists, oncologists or endocrinologists. Few refer to each other's journals, so there is little sense of overall perspective. [90]

Rick Lane makes an important point in showing how today's disease specialization has segmented medical practice and sublimated awareness of the *wholeness* of their patients' various systems. Throughout this book, and others in this Living Superfood series, my aim is to elevate the concept of the body's integration of its systems; that they all work together as a collaborative matrix. Lane writes:

Examining diseases in isolation, medical researchers have historically paid little attention to evolutionary theories, and tend to consider illness from a mechanistic point of view. In the case of heart disease, for example, we know in minute detail how oxidized cholesterol builds up in coronary arteries, producing atherosclerotic plaques, how these plaques rupture, and how thrombosis causes myocardial infarction.... What we are far less certain about is how heart disease relates to other diseases of old age, such as cancer, and whether it is possible to prevent body diseases by targeting a common underlying cause...the closest we have come, in the face of all the advances of modern medicine, is to say 'Eat your greens'; and even then we are not quite sure why. [91]

What the author is referring to is a fairly new field of molecular biology, centered on the *prevention* of disease and disorder, called *Functional Medicine*. The paragraph continues:

---

[90] Ibid, Pgs 214-215
[91] Ibid, Pg 215

This bleak situation is gradually changing. With so much at stake in a graying world, many more researchers are applying themselves squarely to the problem of aging. The field of gerontology is now one of the most fertile in biology, and generates more interest than at any time since the alchemists. At last the dismal mountains of biological and medical evidence are being remodeled into broader, testable theories.

Lane then refers to the main theories of aging that have captured the focus of many researchers in the field.

The two main theories of aging – which we might loosely call the programmed and the stochastic theories – are daily growing closer together. Theories of programmed ageing hold that ageing is programmed in the genes, and is equivalent to other developmental processes such as the growth of the embryo, puberty or menopause. Stochastic theories hold, in contrast, that ageing is essentially an accumulation of wear and tear over a lifetime and is not programmed in the genes. As is so often the case in science, the reality lies somewhere in between, drawing on elements from each theory. We do not know all the answers, and many details are perplexing, but in broad terms I think it is true to say that we do now understand why and how we age...aging is not biologically inevitable, and does not follow a fixed genetic programme – although it is most certainly written in the genes. We shall see in future chapters that oxygen is central not just to ageing and death, but also, through the deepest of connections, to sex and the emergence of gender. [92]

As Lane states, "Ageing, or rather senescence – the loss of function over the years – is not inevitable." *Senescence* is defined as "the state of being old or the process of becoming old." This differs from the molecular biology concept of *apoptosis*, which is defined as "the death of a cell, in any form, mediated by an intracellular program." Thus senescence can

---

[92] Ibid, Pgs 215-216

be a cumulative process brought on by a number of body system malfunctions which might result from environmental stresses (resulting from bad diet, exposure to toxins, accidental injuries, etc.) while on the other hand apoptosis is the process by which a cell's life cycle is determined by its own nucleic DNA and genetic expression.

What I aim to pass on to you, the reader, is that according to our understanding of the "Miracle of Life" as it takes place within the molecular, cellular, organic and systemic order within our bodies, both senescence *and* apoptosis are subject to our mediation and modulation through conscious and disciplined lifestyle practices. Of these various disciplines, the practice of sex as an act of preserving our genetic lineage provokes an introspective that is different than how most of us think about sex. This is where the author's research gets even more interesting for me.

> In natural selection, Darwin's idea is most commonly expressed in the phrase coined by the English philosopher Herbert Spencer: the 'survival of the fittest'. This phrase is often criticized by evolutionary biologists as misleading, as natural selection is concerned not with survival as such, but with reproduction. The individuals that *reproduce* themselves most successfully are most likely to pass on their genes to the next generation. Those that fail to reproduce perish (unless, of course, they live forever). But if we step back for a moment, we can see that there is something to be said for Spencer's misrepresentation. Why on earth do individuals want to reproduce themselves at all? Where does the reproductive imperative come from? ...why do living things want so desperately to reproduce?

> The answer is that only reproduction can ensure survival. All complex matter is eventually destroyed by something. Even mountains are eroded over the aeons. The more complex the structure, the more likely it is to be broken down. Organic matter is fragile and will be shredded by ultraviolet rays or chemical attack sooner or later. Its atoms will be recycled in simpler combinations. Carbon dioxide, being a single molecule, is more stable than DNA. On the other hand, if a

piece of matter happens to have a propensity to replicate itself, for a little while its chances of persisting intact are doubled. It is still only a matter of time before the daughters are destroyed, but if one of the daughter molecules succeeds in replicating itself in the meantime, then the process can continue indefinitely. [93]

At this point, the author goes on to lay out a detailed conceptualization of the difference between two distinct methods of species replication: *reproduction* and *sex*, two words which have seemingly become identical and interchangeable for many of us, but when it comes to biological processes, the two concepts are quite distinct from one another. The first part of our understanding of this distinction begins with a realization that the *rate of replication* has evolutionarily determined key differences which distinguish reproduction from sexual replication.

Given the tendency to destruction, the *rate* of replication is profoundly important. If we assume a steady rate of destruction, then to ensure survival, the rate of replication must surpass the rate of destruction. ...In this sense, immortal refers to a *population* of cells that has the potential to continue dividing indefinitely without becoming senescent... In other words, if the rate of replication fails to surpass the rate of destruction, then the overall population will gradually decline and die out, at least in theory.

...Such attacks take place continuously, in a more-or-less random manner. Unless the damage inflicted undermines the integrity of the cell at one fell swoop, the destruction of proteins and lipids is not necessarily a calamity. Given a suitable supply of energy, they can be replaced, new for old, following instructions in the DNA. The problem comes when the code itself, the DNA, is damaged. If the damage to DNA results in the production of a faulty protein, which is incapable of carrying out a critical function such as the manufacture of other proteins, then the cell will almost certainly die. The

---

[93] Ibid Pgs 216-217

central question in biology is therefore how to maintain the integrity of DNA from generation to generation. [94]

Nick Lane then continues to explain in detail why the rate at which DNA is damaged is directly related to the speed at which the cell, or biological entity, is compelled to replicate itself. Simple organisms are more prone to catastrophic destruction of key parts, thus they have adopted the best means for rapid replication which is *reproduction*. He points out that bacteria can replicate themselves many-fold in such a short period of time that a single reproducing cell can produce millions of copies of itself within a day or even within hours. The process of reproduction is best suited for this accelerated rate of multiplication because the cell is able to replicate itself with complete copies of its DNA along with adaptive RNA coding, splitting itself into two parts and thus double its chances of genetic survival, which is especially important in situations where the organism is under constant danger of annihilation. Lane writes:

This is natural selection at work. Several changes take place in the cells. First of all, some of the cells divide faster. These faster replications are disproportionately represented among the survivors because they are more likely to have replicated themselves before their DNA was destroyed. For the population as a whole, each population doubling now takes place in a shorter period. The survivors produce a new set of genes in a shorter time than that required for radiation to dismember a single set. The progeny now have a greater than 50 percent probability of surviving intact to the next generation.

As long as the cells have sufficient space and nutrients, this adaptation alone might suffice. However, many cells have probably made a second, closely related adaptation. As the population growth steadies, we see that these cells have extra copies of their own DNA. They now have multiple identical chromosomes...if the cell has multiple copies of all its genes, it can take an equivalent number of hits with a good

---

[94] Ibid, Pg 217-218

chance that the *same* gene will not be destroyed on all the chromosomes. [95]

You might be asking, as does the author at this point, "What does all this have to do with aging?" He answers:

> Bacteria, for the most part, do not age. There is no reason for them to do so. They maintain the integrity of their genes by rapid reproduction. They can produce a new generation every 30 minutes. They protect themselves by hoarding multiple chromosomes, by exchanging genes through conjugation and later gene transfer and by fixing damaged DNA whenever possible... Bacteria have behaved in this way for nearly 4 billion years. Certainly they have evolved, and in this sense they have aged, but in every other respect they are as youthful now as they were all those countless generations ago. [96]

Lane then begins to compare the life-replication cycle of bacteria to that of more *evolved* species which have taken on the process of *senescence* (from the Latin: senescere, meaning "to grow old") or "aging" as we commonly refer to the process. This is where distinctions between reproduction and sex, beg further clarification:

> Aging evolved at the same time as sex. By sex (I should come clean) I mean the production of sex cells such as sperm and egg and their fusion to form a new organism. The terms 'sex' and 'reproduction' are often used interchangeably, but technically they have completely different meanings. As John Maynard Smith and Eőrs Szathmáry put it, "the sexual process is in fact the opposite of reproduction. In reproduction, one cell divides into two; in sex, two cells fuse to form one." This poses a puzzle, which we shall see applies as much to aging as to sex: what is the benefit to the individual? [97]

---

[95] Ibid, Pg 218-219
[96] Ibid, Pg 220
[97] Ibid, Pg 221

Lane then goes on to explain that the greatest benefit to sex as a means of replication is that it allows for swift dispersal of advantageous gene mutations throughout an entire population, as well as to allow the process of wider variation within species; one can rarely if ever find two individuals within the world's population of over 7.25 billion people who are exactly alike, except for the case of identical twins. Identical twins, in a manner similar to the replication of bacteria, have formed two entities from a single fertilized egg which has successfully managed to copy its DNA and split into two.

In describing the sex-replication process and how it has become beneficial to humans, even to include evolutionary benefits of aging, he goes on to write:

> For a trait to become established in a population, it must first be beneficial to *individuals*, who then thrive at the expense of other individuals lacking the trait... In sexual reproduction, two robust individuals who have succeeded against the odds to surviving until sexual maturity, and then mating, have their robust genetic constitutions shuffled and recombined into new combinations in the offspring that, in statistical terms, are likely to be less robust... [W]e should just note that the same considerations apply to senescence. If senescence evolved, then it must have been beneficial to individuals or it could never have become such an integral feature of a large part of the living world. Senescence is, in fact, even more widespread than sex, affecting essentially all plants and animals, implying that the advantage must be very pervasive. [98]

I find this research quite compelling and I hope you the reader are able to understand these related topics of senescence (the programmed process of aging), replication, reproduction and sex in the context of our overall goal of extending length and quality of lifespan. There's one more critical point that I'm compelled to share from within this book, which expands established boundaries of our current comprehension of

---

[98] Ibid, Pg 221

biological processes. I feel it necessary to share the following excerpt which helps us to put the concept of "sex" into a radical new perspective:

> The fundamental problem with sex is the *rate* of reproduction. If an asexual microorganism, such as a bacterium, reproduces by simply dividing into two (*binary fusion*), then one cell produces two, two cells produce four and so on. The population as a whole expands at an exponential rate. The rate of sexual propagation is necessarily much slower, two cells conjoin to produce one, and this must, at the very least, divide in two before it can produce daughter cells that can fuse with other cells to produce more offspring. Not only is the rate of reproduction slower, but the sex cells also have to find each other, and determine that they are right for each other, before they can fuse and then reproduce. The process is fraught with danger and is energetically costly. An asexual population should outnumber a sexual population in a handful of generations. Alternatively, if one individual in a sexual population were to revert to asexual reproduction, the asexual progeny should swiftly outnumber the sexual progeny. On the basis of simple arithmetic, sex should never have got started. Having evolved against all the odds, it ought to have been weeded out long ago. [99]

As the author wrote about *asexual* reproduction – the ability of a complex organism to replicate itself without the need for contribution from another member of its own species – I am reminded of the stories in the religious fable of "Immaculate Conception." In our understanding of this research, these two ideas would be equivalent: Immaculate Conception *equals* asexual reproduction. While described as a miraculous event in various descriptions of religious phenomena, we don't have hard evidence of this actually taking place within the human species outside of religious texts. Theoretically, it could be possible as the female DNA, does seemingly have all the necessary seed components to fashion another body, male or female. Yet, like simple bacteria, the complications of self-replicating capacity among females would have likely directed human evolution along a totally different

---

[99] Iid, Pgs 221-222

course – of the likely outcomes would have resulted in a significantly shortened lifespan as well as the possible disappearance of males as an unnecessary factor for sexual replication.

20 Years ago, there was much attention given to the case of "Dolly the Sheep", an experiment involving a cloned sheep, born in July 1996 and touted widely within the media as the practical arrival of species cloning. This announcement provoked quite an impassioned response from all camps, ranging from the hopeful promise of new means for animal husbandry to cries of outrage from those who resented "scientists playing God" and possibly using the same technology to clone humans. I do recall the number of people in the conspiracy circles who claimed that this was already being done with humans, citing different theories on where it was taking place. I remained skeptical about the whole cloning process and these tales from when I first heard of Dolly's birth.

A few years later the follow-up story quietly emerged that the sheep cloning experiment had failed miserably. "**Dolly the sheep dies young**", read the headline of an article in *New Scientist*, in its February 2003 issue. [100] Their story read in part:

> Dolly the sheep, the first mammal to be cloned from an adult cell, was put down on Friday afternoon, after developing a progressive lung disease.

> Dolly's birth six-and-a-half years' ago caused a sensation around the world. But as many sheep live to twice this age, her death will refuel the intense debate over the health and life expectancy of cloned animals.

> The type of lung disease Dolly developed is most common in older sheep. And in January 2002, it was revealed that Dolly had developed arthritis prematurely. She was cloned using a cell taken from a healthy six-year-old sheep, and was born on 5 July 1996 at the Roslin Institute, Edinburgh, Scotland.

> ...Some cloned mammals, including Dolly, have shorter telomeres than other animals of the same age. Telomeres are

---

[100] Dolly the sheep dies young, by Will Knight, from New Scientist, 14 February 2003

pieces of DNA that protect the ends of chromosomes. They shorten as cells divide and are therefore considered a measure of ageing in cells.

As this experiment on cloning mammalian species definitively demonstrated, duplicating whole-chromosome cells from an animal in a *sex-less* manner of replication, mimicking the process of reproduction, produces a shortened lifespan outcome. What the conductors of the experiment learned were that the *programmed senescence* within the DNA of an adult will have created the process by which the cloned offspring itself will represent the same maturation, and degree of senescence, as the clone's parent-cell donor. Reproduction from a single cell duplicating all of its chromosomes to form another copy of its self consistently produces short lifespan. Let the record stand clearly that cloning humans, although it may have been attempted, is doomed to failure because of cellular senescence.

Human sexual replication took a different course than *asexual reproduction*. The splitting of our chromosomes into 23 pairs within the sperm cells, with half potentially encoding xx-chromosome (female) and half, potentially encoding XY-chromosome (male) in the resulting conjunction with the egg. There are asexual animals such as species of crayfish, Komodo Dragons, "all-lady" whiptail lizards, hammerhead sharks, and certain wasps. Some of these species are not *exclusively* asexual but have been known to adapt in certain environments where males of the species were not available.

At this point, I do need to make an important distinction between the shortened lifespan of a cloned mammalian cell and the difference in life expectancy compared to identical twins, themselves resulting from the process of cellular DNA duplication followed by the embryonic cell splitting into two identical copies. The difference here is that the embryonic cell which duplicated itself (producing 96 chromosome pairs before splitting) was the product of *meiosis* (sex replication) – 23 pairs of chromosomes came from each of two opposite-gender members of the same species. This should further confirm our understanding of how the evolution of sex among humans and other species *directly* contributes to longevity in contrast to the process of DNA-duplication and cell-splitting which we can now refer to more accurately as *reproduction*.

The final point I wish to make as I close this chapter is to bring awareness of a profound insight which I've gained from this study of *Oxygen – The Molecule that Made the World*. Our current cultural projection of the idea of "sex" is distorted by widely dispersed ideas, moralities, and social constructs. While we are all likely aware and appalled at the way that "sex" is used to manipulate our psychologies toward control, marketing, and psychic entrapment, in reality, the very common concept of "sex" is itself a distortion of the biological function. To be clear, sex is very necessary for the preservation of the human species and as such, it is biochemically a very powerful incentive incorporating many of the body systems.

Yet, because we can now distinguish the different formations of biological replication which contrast reproduction from sex, we can now understand that sex is the specific process of meiosis, by which complimentary pairings of male and female chromosomes, 23 pairs within the sperm and 23 pairs within the egg, conjoin together in an illustrious dance to form the 46 chromosome pairs which are needed to initiate the process of creating another human being. Thus, if this process fails at any of a number of given points it will not result in successful replication.

We can use our scientific understanding of these processes to facilitate labeling of much of the activity that takes place between humans as *lovemaking* or *copulation,* as opposed to sex-replication. Without going too deeply into what might be interpreted as moralistic proselytizing, we can now put into context the various behaviors that we witness within society and ask certain key questions. Do these acts lead to successful replication of our species? Are the participants aware of the biological profundity of their behaviors? When a society *normalizes* lifestyles that do not promote species survival, is that a truly healthy society?

As well, another surprising question arises as to whether non-asexual, non-replicating members of a species could be expected to experience a longer or shorter lifespan than their replicating fellows? Answering these questions would likely demand the collection and examination of another specialized data set for which I am not herein prepared to pursue. Still, the biological processes of replication, reproduction, and sex do offer us some very interesting points of inquiry and understanding of our quest for high-quality life extension.

# Chapter 18 – **The Value of Exercise in Longevity**

During the extensive 2015 LIBRadio broadcast series that initiated this book on longevity, the scientific insights, lifestyle tips and comprehension of the spectrum of factors which lead to high-quality life extension just kept getting more practicable. By the middle of the month, I was starting to notice physiological effects from applying the insights I was learning. There came a point when it was obvious, from looking at myself in the mirror in the mornings to the way that my flow during my daily broadcast transpired, that access to a renewed level of vital energy had become apparent. I similarly hope that you, by the time you've reached this chapter, are experiencing similar effects.

While a constant stream of advisors has rightly instructed the public as to the value of exercise to a healthy lifestyle, one still wonders just how much exercise is necessary and which types of exercise are best? Answers to both questions need to be better understood.

Professional bodybuilders are a group which obviously engages in far more exercise over the course of their careers than does the general public. While it is not easy to get precise statistics on the average age-of-death for professional bodybuilders, it has been variously reported to being somewhere between 55-58 years-of-age, far less than the average age of death for all men within the United States; 76 years of expected lifespan.

Bodybuilders engage in multiple practices which can be *extremely* stressful on their glandular system, digestion, lipid management, and cardiovascular integrity. As well, bodybuilders display elevated levels of an inflammatory blood marker called *C-Reactive Protein* while they consume a very high-calorie diet, which defies all accepted research on extending life expectancy because it can trigger the redox cascade (promotion of free radicals). An article on health risks from bodybuilding, published in a Zimbabwe newspaper, explained:

"The body uses protein for building the muscles, whilst the carbohydrates provide the large amounts of energy needed to sustain the grueling training. This is known as the bulking phase of training. Once muscle growth has progressed, the athletes may then adjust their method of training to incorporate more sculpting exercises whilst remaining on a high protein, low fat, moderate carbohydrate diet to reduce fat in the body and maintain the muscle gained during the growth/bulking phase."

Bodybuilders who then decide to enter a competition go through a third phase known as the pre-contest preparation phase. ¶ In the few days leading to the contest, salt, water and carbohydrates are severely restricted and eventually eliminated in order to obtain maximum definition. [101]

Many bodybuilders also consume injections and oral supplements of anabolic steroids, along with other "medications synthesized that mimic the effects of the male hormone testosterone in the body," wrote author Brian Nkiwane for the Zimbabwe newspaper *The Standard*. He added that "These drugs do have some immediate side effects that include increased blood pressure, liver stress, temporary shut-down of the body's natural production of male hormones as well as heart-by-pass." One of the main suspected causes of early death among men, and increasingly women, who follow this body-bulking regime for many years, is when they stop taking the medications. Nkiwane wrote further:

"What then causes a short lifespan is that those athletes that take the drugs with the help of medical practitioners always go for professional advice, even when they feel they no longer want to continue using them.

"Their medical advisors then give them other forms of tablets that they take to wean them off properly to avoid side effects. But look what happens with our own athletes; if they decide to stop using drugs, they just wake up the following day not

---

[101] Bodybuilding: The pros and cons, by Brian Nkiwane, from The Standard of Zimbabwe, Jan. 2013

taking them, just like that. All I am saying is that this sudden cut off supply in the body will definitely have side effects".

Another health study compared the Japanese sport of sumo wrestling to professional bodybuilding, pointing out that one common factor among both groups, the high-caloric diets of these athletes, was consistently associated with shortened life expectancy. It reported:

> Despite the beneficial effects of regular exercise, the life expectancy of competitive athletes varies depending on their sport. Phelan and Rose note that high daily caloric intake is linked to reduced life expectancy, with the average male sumo wrestler living an average of 20 years less than the average male. Although this may be due to the higher body fat percentage of sumo wrestlers, the high protein consumption of bodybuilders may have similar effects on life expectancy. As noted by Dr. Joel Fuhrman of Disease Proof, high-protein diets are associated with life expectancies at least 10 years shorter than the North American average. [102]

For the purposes of this chapter concerning the role of exercise toward *high quality* life extension, we engage exercise toward a different outcome than that of bulking up the body, sculpting overall form in order to impress bodybuilding contest judges, turning the body into a massive muscular machine, or putting forward a hyper-masculine image through bulking up. People are considering the value of exercise for their own lifestyle, which might be classified into groups ranging from sedentary to those who regularly engage in high-impact sports. As we shall reveal, the data linking various types and varying amounts of exercise to longevity can be complex, but it is very informative.

There are three types of exercise that are generally recommended for ultimate health and, accordingly, extended lifespan and quality of life; they are 1) cardiovascular, 2) strength training, and 3) stretch/balance. During the process which initiated this book, I was able to digest a large collection of studies, research articles, and position papers from health advocates on these various types of exercise individually, as well as the

---

[102] Sumo Wrestlers Compared to Bodybuilders, by Matthew Lee, LiveStrong.com, July 2015

overall impact of exercise on longevity outcome. I will share some of the highlights from this set of analyses.

Before we segment exercise into these three categories, let's first establish a level of overall exercise which has proved complementary to this goal of high-quality life extension.

The *New York Times* posted an article by Gretchen Reynolds, "**The Right Dose of Exercise for a Longer Life**," [103] which cited two recent studies in the *Journal of the American Medical Association (JAMA) Internal Medicine*, one of which originated from the National Cancer Institute in partnership with Harvard University and other institutions. Reynolds, citing this particular study, noted certain key findings:

- "[T]he researchers stratified the adults by their weekly exercise time, from those who did not exercise at all to those who worked out for 10 times the current recommendations or more (meaning that they exercised moderately for 25 hours per week or more). Then they compared 14 years' worth of death records for the group. They found that, unsurprisingly, the people who did not exercise at all were at the highest risk of early death."

- "Those who met the guidelines precisely, completing 150 minutes per week of moderate exercise, enjoyed greater longevity benefits and 31 percent less risk of dying during the 14-year period compared with those who never exercised."

- "The sweet spot for exercise benefits, however, came among those who tripled the recommended level of exercise, working out moderately, mostly by walking, for 450 minutes per week, or a little more than an hour per day. Those people were 39 percent less likely to die prematurely than people who never exercised."

- "At that point, the benefits plateaued, the researchers found, but they never significantly declined. Those few individuals engaging in 10 times or more the recommended exercise dose gained about the same reduction in mortality risk as people who simply met the guidelines."

---

[103] The Right Dose of Exercise for a Longer Life, by Gretchen Reynolds, The New York Times, April 2015

Other research correlated the length of time spent exercising to an expected outcome in stretching lifespan. Author Carey Goldberg, writing a blog for Boston NPR radio affiliate WBUR, talked about the federal guidelines for 150 minutes of exercise per week and the struggle that people had to achieve such lifestyle habits. He cites findings from a major published research study that put direct reward-to-input ratios on what life extension benefits one should expect from a commitment to regular exercise. Goldberg's article, entitled "**Every Minute of Exercise Could Lengthen Your Life Seven Minutes**," shares with us the findings of a peer review journal publication; essentially summarizing the conclusion of the studies in its very title. Goldberg's article is itself inspiring and informative. The title of the referenced research study, published online from *PLOS Journals*, was a bit less direct, entitled "**Leisure Time Physical Activity of Moderate to Vigorous Intensity and Mortality: A Large Pooled Cohort Analysis.**"

Few of us are attracted to peer review journals because the degree of literacy needed to wade through the scientific jargon used within these publications can often be daunting. I have developed the skills to plod through these studies over many years. I began reading this literature from right after high school when I found my first (and only so far) career job working in a laboratory in the field of reproductive biology. Here's an example of moderately cryptic medical journal writing, from this aforementioned PLOS-published article, to illustrate this challenge:

> We examined the association of leisure time physical activity with mortality during follow-up in pooled data from six prospective cohort studies in the National Cancer Institute Cohort Consortium, comprising 654,827 individuals, 21–90 y of age. Physical activity was categorized by metabolic equivalent hours per week (MET-h/wk). Life expectancies and years of life gained/lost were calculated using direct adjusted survival curves (for participants 40+ years of age), with 95% confidence intervals (CIs) derived by bootstrap. The study includes a median of 10 y of follow-up and 82,465 deaths. A physical activity level of 0.1–3.74 MET-h/wk, equivalent to brisk walking for up to 75 min/wk, was associated with a gain of 1.8 (95% CI: 1.6–2.0) y in life expectancy relative to no leisure time activity (0 MET-h/wk). Higher levels of physical

activity were associated with greater gains in life expectancy, with a gain of 4.5 (95% CI: 4.3–4.7) y at the highest level (22.5+ MET-h/wk, equivalent to brisk walking for 450+ min/wk). Substantial gains were also observed in each BMI group. In joint analyses, being active (7.5+ MET-h/wk) and normal weight (BMI 18.5–24.9) was associated with a gain of 7.2 (95% CI: 6.5–7.9) y of life compared to being inactive (0 MET-h/wk) and obese (BMI 35.0+). A limitation was that physical activity and BMI were ascertained by self report.

From which the 14 authors of the study offered up a much simplified concluding statement:

More leisure time physical activity was associated with longer life expectancy across a range of activity levels and BMI groups. [104] [BMI stands for body mass index]

Another of our favorite online sources for practical information that is both well researched as well as paradigm challenging is the noted health researcher Dr. Joseph Mercola. His popular online forum is claimed to be the "world's #1 natural health website." As a great go-to online resource for all things healthy, his perspective regarding the close association between regular exercise and longevity should be useful for our analysis. In an article entitled, "How Exercise Can Help You Live Longer", Mercola wrote:

One of the key things you can do to extend not only the quantity of your years, but also the quality, is to make a few simple changes to your lifestyle. One of the most important changes is regulating your insulin and leptin levels through diet and exercise.

I've often stated that your diet accounts for about 80 percent of the benefits you'll reap from a healthy lifestyle, but even if

---

[104] Leisure Time Physical Activity of Moderate to Vigorous Intensity and Mortality: A Large Pooled Cohort Analysis / November 6, 2012, http://dx.doi.org/10.1371/journal.pmed.1001335

you're eating the best diet in the world, you still need to exercise effectively to reach your highest level of health.

This means incorporating core-strengthening exercises, strength training, stretching, and high-intensity activities into your rotation. High-intensity interval training boosts human growth hormone (HGH) production, which is essential for optimal health, strength, vigor, and yes—longevity. [105]

One of the hallmarks of modern society is that people are spending more of their day in sedentary activity than at any other time in history. Because of the information age, many spend the bulk of their working day at a desk, fixed to a computer screen, only to drive home to spend long hours parked in front of the television or otherwise inactive. Our ancestors spent many more hours of the day engaged in hunter-gatherer activities or getting physical exercise through agricultural labor or more physical industrial productivity. This modern sedentary lifestyle has now become so closely associated with poor health outcome that it is being referred to as "the new cigarette smoking" as it impacts people's health. Mercola stated in the article:

> That said, intermittent movement is equally (if not more) critical for maximizing the quality of your life. Chronic, undisrupted sitting—even if you maintain an optimum fitness program—has been found to be an independent risk factor for premature death. Intermittent movement is nothing more than the interruption of sitting, which can be done simply by standing up every 15 minutes or so. Physical activity also produces biochemical changes that strengthen and renew your brain—particularly areas associated with memory and learning.

The online article recommends five types of exercise necessary for optimal fitness:

1.  Interval (anaerobic) training – short bursts of high-intensity exercise and recovery;

---

[105] How Exercise Can Help You Live Longer, by Dr. Mercola, May 02, 2014 / Mercola.com

2. Strength training – using weights to reinforce muscular and bone strength;

3. Core exercises – working out the muscles located in your back, abdomen, and pelvis;

4. Stretching – to improve circulation and increase the elasticity of muscle joints;

5. Stand up every 15 minutes – efforts to keep the body moving all day long.

One of the most effective means of getting the right amount and type of cardiovascular conditioning, which Dr. Mercola claims as among his favorite techniques, is *high-intensity interval training (HIIT)*. On that technique he wrote:

> I've often stated that to optimize your benefits from exercise, you'll want to push your body hard enough for a challenge, while still allowing adequate time for recovery and repair. One of the best ways to accomplish this is with high-intensity interval training (HIIT), which consists of short bursts of high-intensity exercise followed by longer periods of recovery, as opposed to extended episodes of continuous vigorous exertion. This is a core part of my Peak Fitness program, and the Australian study makes a case for the wisdom of such an approach.

My own experience also highlights the value of high-intensity interval training exercise. I can invest 20 minutes 4-6 days a week in this activity. I will walk vigorously for 90 seconds and then spend 30 seconds running at the fastest pace my respiration can tolerate. I use a stopwatch to time this cycle accurately. After the 30-second burst, I cool down while walking briskly and the 90 seconds interval seems to restore me sufficiently to take off running again. I repeat this two-minute-cycle ten times, five out and an additional five back toward home. This is pretty invigorating and challenging. I do caution people to work up to HIIT and don't try to hit your peak on the first day or even the first week. It can be very stressful on underused muscles and joints.

Additionally, and this is very important, like so many studies found throughout the medical literature, Mercola points out the critical importance of regular exercise to maintain optimal brain, memory and cognitive functioning, which is known to degrade as we age:

> As discussed in a recent post, obesity is associated with cognitive decline, in part because it increases levels of inflammatory chemicals known as cytokines in your body, which are strongly damaging to brain function. According to a study published in the *Journal of Neuroscience,* it appears your body may react to excess fat as an invader, causing levels of cytokines to stay elevated, thereby causing chronic inflammation.
>
> Exercise is, of course, a key ingredient for weight loss. But it's also a simple yet remarkably potent way to lower your levels of inflammatory cytokines, which will help protect your brain function.
>
> Physical exercise has also been found to protect against other age-related brain changes. For example, those who exercise the most tend to have the least amount of brain shrinkage over time. Not only that, but exercise actually causes your brain to *grow* in size. For example, Kirk I. Erickson, PhD of the University of Pittsburgh found that adults aged 60 to 80 who walked for 30 to 45 minutes, three days per week for one year, showed a two percent increase in the volume of their hippocampus — a brain region associated with memory.

Further recommendations from Chicago-based fitness trainer Val Walkowiak, for *4 Simple Strength-Training Exercises* which should be engaged every other day, were cited in an online article from Everyday Health website, written by Wyatt Myers. [106] Let's share what sounds like very reasonable recommendations:

- **Abdominal Twist:** "Sit in an armless chair with your feet flat on the floor and shoulder-width apart. Your hands should be in the center

---

[106] 4 Muscle-Building Exercises for Aging Gracefully, By Wyatt Myers from EveryDayHealth.com

of your torso and your elbows along your sides. Slowly twist to the right, then to the left. Your shoulders should face to the right and then to the left during the movement, but you should not be swinging your arms from side to side. Do two to three sets of 15 to 20 repetitions."

- **Lying Abdominal Crunch**: "Lie on your back with your legs bent and your feet flat on the floor. Place your hands by your ears. Keep your elbow and shoulder joints aligned during the movement. Slowly curl your upper body upward until your ribcage comes up off the floor. The goal is to create a "C" with your torso by bringing your chest toward your legs. Don't let your lower back come up off the floor, just your rib cage. Perform two to three sets of 15 to 20 repetitions."

- **Pelvic Tilts**: "Lie on your back with your legs bent and feet flat on the floor. Pull your belly button in toward your spine until your abdominal muscles feel tight. Slowly shift your pelvis up toward the ceiling until you feel your lower back pressed against the floor. Your buttocks should not come off the floor. Return to starting position. This exercise works the lower portion of the abdominal muscles."

- **Bridges**: "Lie on your back with your legs bent and feet flat on the floor. Pull your belly button in toward your spine. Slowly lift your torso off the floor until you have formed a bridge with your body. Your upper back, shoulders, and head should remain on the floor. Return your body to the floor and repeat. Perform two to three sets of 15 to 20 repetitions."

Toward our goal of increased quality and extension of life, the benefits to be gained from stress-reducing exercise are also very important. Stress can be a critical factor that inhibits optimal function for most of our body systems. Hormonal secretions associated with stress can result in hypertension, stroke, sleep disorders, digestive problems, altered reproductive functioning, headache, fatigue, muscle tension, and chest pain. Additionally, mental problems associated with stress hormone buildup include depression and anxiety.

To say the least, a major component of our healthy longevity program should include stress-reducing exercise. Taken from an article by Beth Orenstein, writing for Everyday Health, we have 8 recommendations for optimal health, exercise and stress relief. Her article began with the following note:

> Exercise is one of the best ways to reduce stress. "When you exercise, your body releases endorphins, which are hormones that fight stress," says Frank Lupin, MS, ATC, PES, a certified athletic trainer and a personal trainer for Coordinated Health in Bethlehem, Pa. "Exercise helps you get your mind off your problems and clears your head," adds Thomas Plante, PhD, an associate professor of psychology at Santa Clara University in California. Here are eight different kinds of exercise that can heighten energy and provide stress relief. [107]

Orenstein's 8 recommendations for stress-reducing exercise follow:

- **High-Energy Activities** – "The benefits of aerobic exercise — like running, dancing, spinning, and in-line roller-skating — include an increased heart rate. When your heart rate is accelerated, your body releases endorphins, natural opiates that make you feel good with no side effects."

- **Yoga** – "an excellent stress-relief exercise, involves a series of moving and stationary poses, or postures, combined with deep breathing. For stress relief, do gentle yoga or yoga for beginners — popular "power yoga" classes may be too intense if your main goal is to ease stress."

- **Tai Chi** – "According to recent studies, Tai chi can help build bone density, lower blood pressure, boost the immune system, and even ease symptoms of conditions like heart failure, arthritis, and fibromyalgia. Another advantage is that it is an easy activity for people of all ages to incorporate into everyday life."

- **Pilates** – Are "a series of controlled movements and mat exercises designed to build your strength, flexibility, and endurance — all of which makes practicing Pilates an anaerobic (as opposed to aerobic) exercise, a great stress reliever. Pilates also tones your body."

---

[107] Exercise and Stress Relief, By Beth W. Orenstein, published at EverydayHealth.com

- **Martial Arts** – "Are another effective way to release energy, frustration, and tension. There are many to choose from. In addition, martial arts have other benefits; they teach you self-discipline, and the self-defense techniques you learn can make you feel safer."

- **Kickboxing** – "This involves controlled punching and kicking movements carried out with discipline. Kickboxing regularly will help improve your balance, flexibility, and coordination. It's also a great way to work out frustration; having an outlet to release anger can relieve stress."

- **Team Sports** – "You get a double dose of stress relief from participating in team sports: Not only are you having fun with loved ones, but you're also working up a sweat and releasing endorphins. Exercising with friends or co-workers can also motivate you to stay competitive."

- **Take It on the Road** – "Long-distance running, biking, cross-country skiing, and other outdoor activities provide a change of scenery and a dose of fresh air, both of which can help clear your mind. Also, beautiful settings, especially in spring and fall, can lift your mood and shake up your workout routine."

When we incorporate regular exercise into our habitual routines, involving cardio-workout, strength-training, and stretch/balance exercise, we are able to engage actively, directly under our control, that we can be assured will add quality years to our lifespan as it also creates a spectrum of brain and mood advantages. Our longevity goal involves integrating and balancing the mind, body, and spirit. I trust that these suggestions will serve you as well as they have served me on your journey toward mastery of all of the avenues for high-quality life extension.

# Chapter 19 – **Our Need for Sleep and the Hormone Melatonin**

At this point, our trek towards the goal of healthy longevity brings us to the critical need for sleep. How much sleep do we need? What is quality sleep? What is our current state of understanding about the pineal gland, our brain's agent for synchronizing with the circadian rhythm? And what is the long-term impact of disrupted sleep cycles on our overall health?

We can begin this analysis by pointing out the critical role of the hormone *melatonin*, which is secreted by the pineal gland. Melatonin is highly engaged as one of the most powerful endocrine agents for healthy functioning within our glandular system. In this chapter, we will demonstrate why there is also quite likely a need for most people to supplement their nutrition with melatonin if their goal is to extend quality life-years.

Earlier in this book, we examined the rising epidemic of *metabolic syndrome*, a collection of disorders related to malfunctioning within the body's metabolism. Metabolic hormones are produced and utilized all throughout the body and are vitally important endogenous chemicals (manufactured by the body) which regulate a variety of systemic functions. Inability to properly manufacture and manage metabolic hormones, which are regulated by glandular controllers such as the pituitary and thyroid glands, inevitably will lead to serious consequences resulting in disease, disorder, and shortened lifespan. What is very important to the proper functioning of the metabolic glandular system is getting adequate sleep; failing to do so has been linked to several disorders.

*Respiratory Medicine Journal* published the results of a study examining the consequences of two sleep disorders, *obstructive sleep apnea (OSA)* and *excessive daytime sleepiness (EDS)*. The study examined the impact that inadequate sleep had on blood plasma levels of neuropeptides (short-chain, protein-like molecules which are used by neurons to communicate with each other) and metabolic hormones. Throughout this chapter, we will emphasize just how important these particular elements are to our optimized body functioning. This brief conclusion from this study publication entitled **"Plasma levels of neuropeptides and metabolic hormones, and sleepiness in obstructive sleep apnea,"** is very informative:

> Our study shows that EDS in patients with OSA is associated with increased circulating hypocretin-1 and decreased circulating ghrelin levels, two peptides involved in the regulation of body weight, energy balance, sympathetic tone and sleep-wake cycle. This relationship is independent of AHI [apnea-hypopnea index] and obesity (two key phenotypic features of OSA). [108]

While this article points to associated negative outcomes from sleep-deprived plasma hormone levels, relative to the regulation of conditions such as deregulation of body weight (*ghrelin* is one of the main hormones to stimulate hunger; levels of this hormone increase before meals and decrease after meals), energy imbalance, malfunction of the feedback system between body organs and the central nervous system (sympathetic tone, related to communication within the body) and management of the *circadian rhythm*, our brain's ability to biochemically distinguish day from night.

From the online publication *Healthline,* we highlight an article, **"The Effects of Sleep Deprivation on the Body,"** written by Ann Pietrangelo. In it the author offered a long list of disorders which have been linked to sleep deprivation, including: improper brain function affecting cognitive integrity and emotional stability; interference with balance, coordination, and decision-making abilities; amplified effects of alcohol consumption and increased susceptibility to accidents; along with multiple disturbances of the central nervous system as well as other body systems involving immune, respiratory, digestive, energy management and cardiovascular functions. Pietrangelo wrote:

> When you're deprived of sleep, your brain can't function properly, affecting your cognitive abilities and emotional

---

[108] Plasma levels of neuropeptides and metabolic hormones, and sleepiness in obstructive sleep apnea. / Respiratory Medicine 2011 Dec;105(12):1954-60

state. If it continues long enough, it can lower your body's defenses, putting you at risk of developing chronic illness. The more obvious signs of sleep deprivation are excessive sleepiness, yawning, and irritability. Chronic sleep deprivation can interfere with balance, coordination, and decision-making abilities. You're at risk of falling asleep during the day, even if you fight it. Stimulants like caffeine are not able to override your body's profound need for sleep. [109]

Brain function and mood are very much a consequence of the constant interplay between a vast spectrum of hormonal and neurological processes. With regard to proper sleep management, we can identify a few key parts of this sleep/wake cycle complex that need to be understood by anyone who wishes to take a positive and interactive role in directing their health, to include the body's autonomous systems regulation (the 90% of our brain function outside of our conscious control). By the mere act of achieving an optimized sleep cycle pattern, we can then provide a foundation for the best outcome with regard to the spectrum of body maintenance activities which we earlier cited as being negatively impacted by sleep deprivation. Let's identify a few of these components of the sleep/wake cycle with the intention of using our understanding toward creating the right conditions for each stage to contribute toward our optimal health.

- **Somnolence** – "Similar to drowsiness, somnolence occurs when a person has a strong desire for sleep. It is also a term that is used to describe excessive sleepiness during the day and certain sleep disorders. For most people, drowsiness at bedtime is a natural part of the circadian rhythm, although excessive tiredness and daytime sleepiness could be a sign of a sleep disorder." [110]

- **Pineal gland** – "Both melatonin and its precursor, serotonin, which are derived chemically from the alkaloid substance tryptamine, are synthesized in the pineal gland. Along with other brain sites, the pineal gland may also produce neurosteroids...though the

---

[109] The Effects of Sleep Deprivation on the Body, Written by Ann Pietrangelo, August 19, 2014 / HealthLine.com
[110] What is Somnolence?, by Lindsay Woolman, from LoveToKnow.com

conclusion by 17th-century French philosopher René Descartes that the pineal gland is the seat of the soul has endured as a historical curiosity, there is no evidence to support the notion that secretions from the pineal have a major role in cognition... ¶ Relatively little is known about genetic variants that influence melatonin levels and the relationship of those variants to sleep disorders and other circadian pathologies. Nonetheless, melatonin administration has been associated with numerous and diverse effects, including immune responses, cellular changes, and protection against oxidative stress." [111]

- **Circadian rhythm** – This is the brain and body's synchronization with solar cycles. With the onset of nighttime, unless our sleep patterns are disturbed by outside forces (bright lights, television, electronic activity, social media, etc.), our brains are increasingly bathed with melatonin, thus signaling that the time for sleep has arrived. With the arrival of sunrise, at the end of sleep time which can range from 6-9 hours in the average healthy adult, the hormone dopamine signals that it is time to awaken, and calls the body to action. Children have a greater need for sleep while senior adults will naturally decrease sleep hours as the body ages, a factor which could reasonably be associated with age-related decline in metabolic hormone production.

- **Melatonin** – This hormonal substance, which has such a powerful impact throughout the body, is manufactured by the pineal gland. As dietary supplement melatonin has been called "a longevity hormone" and in numerous studies is clinically indicated to counter Alzheimer's, Parkinson's and Huntington's diseases, regulate weight management and to prevent osteoporosis. Melatonin is also a powerful antioxidant that protects against heart damage and other cardiovascular disease (CVD) conditions, is an immune regulator and cancer treatment booster, and is also very useful for preventing diabetes along with diabetes-associated conditions such as retinopathy (eye damage) and nephropathy (kidney damage). [112]

---

[111] Pineal Gland, written by Charles H. Emerson, Encyclopaedia Britannica
[112] Beyond Sleep: 7 Ways Melatonin Attacks Aging Factors, By Claudia Kelley, PHD, RD, CDE, September 2012

- **Dopamine** – This powerful brain hormone is associated with stimulation, the body's call to action, and is the principal agent which displaces melatonin at the end of the sleep cycle, allowing us to wake (hopefully) refreshed and excited to take on the new day. Other critical functions linked to this "feel-good brain chemical" include motivation, creativity, and impulsivity. Dopamine serves as one of our primary "call to action" hormones.

In addition to melatonin supplements, there are a number of food sources and dietary supplements which can assist us to get the right quality of sleep necessary to achieve optimal health and longevity. Here are just a few of the top sleep supplemental assistants, according to Constance Matthiessen, writing on the topic of "Natural Sleep Aids":

- **Valerian** – "Most experts recommended this herb to reduce the amount of time it takes to nod off...the NIH reports that valerian seems to have sedative properties, and it may increase the amount of GABA (gamma-aminobutyric acid), a compound in the brain that prevents the transmission of nerve impulses. Valerian seems to be especially effective when combined with hops."

- **5-HTP (5-Hydroxytryptophan)** – "A compound derived from the amino acid L-tryptophan, the supplement also is used to enhance mood and decrease appetite... A small 2009 study of 18 people found that those who took a product combining 5-HTP and GABA needed less time to fall asleep, slept longer and reported improved sleep quality."

- **Magnesium** – "Along with contributing to a good night's sleep, this light, the silvery metallic element is an oft-overlooked nutrient that helps maintain normal muscle and nerve function, keeps heart rhythm steady, supports a healthy immune system, and keeps bones strong. Magnesium also helps regulate blood sugar levels and promotes normal blood pressure, according to the NIH [National Institutes of Health]. Lack of magnesium inhibits nerve cell communication, which leads to cell excitability. The result: a stressed and nervous person. Several older studies show that magnesium can improve sleep quality and reduce nocturnal awakenings."

- **Theanine** – "An amino acid derivative found in green tea, theanine has long been known to trigger the release in the brain of gamma-aminobutyric acid, or GABA. GABA activates the major calming neurotransmitters, promoting relaxation and reducing anxiety."

- **Chamomile tea** – Chamomile "is a traditional herbal remedy that has been used since ancient times to fight insomnia and a wide range of other health complaints. Chamomile is sold in the form of tea, extract, and topical ointment... Chamomile's effectiveness as a sleep aid has not been widely researched in humans, but in animal studies, it has been shown to be a safe and mild sleep aid."

Finally, there are multiple techniques that one can easily incorporate that facility healthy sleeping, especially if combating insomnia is the challenge. These include: going to bed and rising at exact, precise times of the day; remove television and computers from the bedroom and turning off electronics at a set time before retiring; limiting the time spent in bed (don't oversleep); using hypnotism or some other cognitive therapy; using guided imagery and meditation techniques; and controlling physiological factors with biofeedback. [113]

There is just no escaping the fact that synchronizing our bodies with the circadian rhythm of day and night is key to making the most of our rest and rejuvenation cycle. Sleep is a critically important component of our quest for quality health and expanded life expectancy. The complex interplay of brain structures, the glandular system, our nutritional patterns and need for avoidance of environmental stressors needs to be brought to full awareness. It is my sincere hope that this collection of insights becomes of great practical use for you as you master the possibilities of high-quality life extension.

---

[113] Coping With Excessive Sleepiness: Natural Sleep Aids, by Constance Matthiessen, from WebMd.com

# Chapter 20 – **Why Live Longer?**

## Loving Our Mothers

As I write today, it is the nation's annual celebration of Mother's Day. For me, this beautiful holiday is somewhat bittersweet because of my own unique family history. My paternal grandmother died long before I entered this world; my father having been the youngest of her nine children. My maternal grandmother had apparently abandoned her only child while still an infant, leaving her in the care of a young husband, a coal miner in the mountains of West Virginia, who was greatly assisted in raising "Peaches" by his brother-in-law's family. Thus, I don't recall ever seeing my only living grandmother until her reappearance for my mother's funeral; Peaches having died much too young at 30 years-of-age, leaving behind a young husband to raise their four sons, including me and my 7-year-old twin.

We were very fortunate to have our maternal grandfather move into our rural home within a community of 21 newly-built homes. There we six males enjoyed the most challenging and rewarding collection of adventures, overshadowed and somewhat haunted by the absence of our mother's love and intimacy. When our father did start dating again, we enjoyed the lovely ladies that he brought into our lives. Within our close-knit neighborhood, there were also spectacular mothers and grandmothers who sympathized with our situation and made it a point to show these four sons much kindness and affection.

As I matured into an adult and ventured out into the world, reverence for women, motherhood, courting-age ladies, grandmothers and all things reflecting the *feminine mystery*, seemed to resonate from a sacred place within my soul. It was as if the spirit of my Goddess Mother was always present in my life's affairs, watching over me, guiding me towards appropriate choices, and making sure that I should always be cognizant of the many feminine expressions of life. Except for those first beautiful 7 years of early life, I've only known my mother in spirit.

What becomes of a child that knows not her or his mother? Can that child ever feel balanced, satisfied, loved and truly in harmony with the larger society?

For me, it took many years to put all of this into a comprehensible context and I can still detect patterns within my life that reflect this imbalance, this unconscious longing for the secure embrace of a mother's love.

I suggest that the same question applies when it comes to loving Mother Earth. This planet embodies the great feminine principle that *is* Life and is embodied in the sacredness of Nature and the idea of a nurturing planet.

Who among us, in their right mind, would *not* strive for healthy longevity for their own birth mother or such for our collective mothers? Gratitude and appreciation for mothers, grandmothers, great-grandmothers and all senior matriarchs are incorporated within the most fundamental and archetypical values of all truly civilized societies. Yet, within America, as well as in other parts of the world, something contradictory has been steadily rising over the span of our generation. The sense of sacredness which is the essence of motherhood is being displaced by something sinister that has risen to prey upon all vulnerable segments of society.

Today our *Great Mother Goddess*, this spirit of motherhood, is being "manhandled" and abused. She is being exploited for her vulnerabilities in pursuit of obscene motives. In the last century hundreds of thousands of mothers, or *would-be* mothers, were illicitly sterilized within sinister, genocidal eugenics campaigns. Within this United States of America, there arose a contemptuous spirit that has maliciously undermined the sanctity of motherhood, resulting in as many as 1.2 million abortions per year within the last decade. The rising cost of living has become so stressing for so many households that mothers are being forced to put their tiny infants into corporate-franchised daycare centers (CAFO's for preschoolers) where babies grow up more dependent on group management systems than the secure intimacy of their own mother's devoted attention.

Who among us would not wish something better for our mothers?

I extend this sentiment of misplaced compassion to our Great Mother; you may prefer to use Mother Nature, some call her the "Great Mother Goddess." I would think that we all have a general valuation of the critical role in every aspect of life's processes that this feminine spirit plays. As such, all women are a reflection of this divine motherhood and we should wish all women the best that society would have to offer, that to include optimal health and longevity.

One of the key motives for a long and productive lifespan is to have something greater-than-self to live for. Realizing one's own *Massive Transforming Purpose (MTP)* in life is an incredibly motivating force. It drives your creativity, causes you to wake up early and stay up late, offers a sense of satisfaction to often-difficult tasks, and will attract a constant stream of others into your life that share your values and are ready to share the journeys we engage throughout life.

An MTP keeps us mentally engaged and physically fit to pursue our dreams, even long after the age by which society encourages us to "retire." Those who have this driving sense of purpose quite often continue to create needed positions for themselves during this retirement phase of their life; working as consultants to growing businesses or volunteering for some public service agencies.

We love to encounter such people in our community or work activities because they often exude a deeply wise and spiritual nature. We are naturally drawn to want to be of special service to these wise elders, to supply their needs for comfort and offer a warm embrace to let them know that we do regard them as special. Our compassionate nature extends this special love to the wise and esteemed elders of our society, our nation, and the world. As we envision our own graceful aging, we long to be revered by the community around us as well.

Yet, increasingly we are seeing the elderly being confined to what amounts to CAFO's for the aging. A vast collection of health-related, profit-driven corporations is cashing in on epidemics of dementia, Alzheimer's and Parkinson's diseases, a spectrum of cognitive disorders, as well as physical disabilities that are increasingly affecting large segments of the senior population. As we are seeing the average life expectancy increase for nearly every nation on Earth, we are correspondingly witnessing the increase of pharmaceutical drug dependence among the elderly. This pandemic is driven by a tidal wave of diagnoses of chronic diseases and increases in financial burdens associated with unhealthy aging. As well, the malicious exploitation of natural aging as a source of profit is being taken advantage of by unrighteous predators of all sorts.

We hate to see our elderly being misused by religious hustlers – selling to the aged the promise of "eternal life in heaven" at a time when many elders increasingly feel anxious about their own impending mortality. Insurance companies and predatory lending agencies similarly have developed special programs offered up to the retired and elderly that, should one examine the fine print of the contracted service, is really just another way of gnawing away at the wealth, or a portion thereof, which should naturally have gone forward to empower a younger generation.

Throughout this book as well as in the lectures and workshops I frequently conduct, I charge that we are witnessing the growth of malicious industries that are profiteering from our many sufferings. This exploitation by the medical industries has gone so far as to making natural aging appear more like a disease, for which they are all too glad to serve up drug solutions at an ever-increasing cost. Turn on an evening television news broadcast and you may likely notice the frequency of pharmaceutical drug advertisements that support programs which are generally more watched by older members of the population. These advertisements are deceptive in that they pretend to offer relief to commonly-experienced health challenges, yet they can barely disguise the potential harm that these medications can cause to the patient. Often the so-called *side effects* of these medications are worse than the original ailment. As well, we often later learn from follow up analysis that these prescribed drugs actually *cause* the disorder to worsen.

You wouldn't do this to a mother you love, would you? How can we tolerate a vast national enterprise that targets our mothers and fathers, grandmothers and grandfathers for such malicious exploitation? How can we accept that media and regulatory agencies allow hundreds of thousands of our venerated elders to be killed or injured each year through malpractice, medical errors, adverse drug reactions, failed therapies and infections of deadly antibiotic-resistant superbugs?

I imagine that you, like me, want to enjoy a long life in part so that we can have time to make things right – to make America (or any other nation we live in or have empathy for) great again. We want to live long in order to see our children, grandchildren, great-grandchildren and their own progeny grow up to be wise, self-motivated, confident and competent in every aspect of being good and productive citizens of the world. We want to live long so that we can bear witness to the transfer of sustainable empowerment to generations so that they can work toward an equitable future. We want to live long in order to amass knowledge and wisdom and to see such wisdom utilized for the benefit of our global family.

Loving our Great Mother is key to survival on this planet. Embracing Nature, in her multiple manifestations, is a bridge to sustainability. One's Massive Transforming Purpose could be to mature into a love that is unlimited, divine, profound and empathetic, and to keep spreading that love every day in every imaginable way. One of my great pleasures in life is to share kind words with the strangers with whom I interact daily. Love is one exercise for which there is never exhaustion. Sharing empathy, kindness, and an authentic compliment are gifts that replenish themselves every time they are given away to others. Laughter and joy, as currency, makes one even richer as this wealth is freely distributed.

Having this vision constantly active within our perceptual awareness is one of the most valuable keys to life. I have offered up my own scientific acumen throughout this book toward the aim of sharing with all who would receive these gifts of knowledge regarding longevity and healthy living.

Senescence (aging) is a natural part of the sacred journey of Life. We should thus not only welcome our maturation but embrace it and make it something valuable within our sacred cosmic journey. Along that journey, we seek to train and discipline ourselves to maintain the most productive habits and lifestyle choices. When one calculates that something is helpful or harmful to our self-interests, we can logically and reasonably adjust our behaviors to take advantage of such revelations that come our way.

When we are able to generously share the joys of our own personal journey through this beautiful life, beautiful Earth and universe full of beauty and wonder, then we are not just living – we are passing on a treasured legacy.

Live long, love strong and prosper, Dear Friend.

# Appendix 1 – **Longevity Gap: Geography & Ethnicity**

Throughout this study, we have had a chance to consider a wide spectrum of topics and issues that can contribute toward healthy aging and life extension. One often overlooked area of investigation is how residential location is also a factor influencing health and lifespan. Here, we look at data that compares how geographic location impacts our chances for longevity. Among the many factors which do have a direct impact on this healthy outcome, directly tied to one's residential environment, are of course wealth and income.

Wealthy people have access to higher quality nutrition, better full-service supermarkets, easier access to healthcare services, emergency facilities, outpatient clinics, exercise facilities, as well as community education, better infrastructure, newer water and sanitation systems, playgrounds, parks, less stressful transportation, as well as better access to localized support services, especially those serving the aging.

There is perhaps no clearer perception of this longevity gap between rich and poor than the data showing the income gap among the world's population overall. There is a tremendous discrepancy in the longevity outcome between the richest nations and the poorest. Many of these same issues of nutrition, access to healthcare clinics, hygiene, sanitation, water, and stress-reducing opportunities are exaggerated even more as the wealth and income gap expands. This is not to curse or condemn those who are born within emerging nations. In certain aspects these residents can have access to better *natural* exercise, a less-processed food diet, clean air, healthy disciplines as well as a strong sense of family, belonging and community support.

Likewise, in most cases, urban residents can be expected to live longer than those in rural areas. There haven't been a lot of studies on the topic, but one can find data that examines health outcomes based upon gender, ethnicity, socioeconomic factors, and level of education as well as urban, suburban or rural differences. One such study, which was published in the *American Journal of Preventive Medicine,* showed overall changes across the U.S. from 1970 to 2009, representing a gain in life expectancy of nearly 8 years but that the lifespan gap favoring urban over rural populations had widened from .4% in 1970 to 2% by 2009.    Factors which contributed to this widening gap included accidents, heart disease, lung conditions, and cancer, as well as higher rates of smoking and obesity.

To the contrary, for Blacks in the U.S., this trend comparing urban to rural is reversed, with rural living favoring the higher life expectancy, especially for males. While poverty rates for rural Blacks were even higher than those of urban residents, the high mortality rate among urban dwellers ran contrary to the national longevity trend.  One study pointed out that a third of black youth would not be expected to survive to 65, mostly due to high rates of chronic diseases, cardiovascular and cancer.  As well, a high rate of mortality among young urban males did factor in as well but it was not the leading factor for the urban discrepancy.

# Appendix 2 – The Impact of Colon Health on Longevity

Colon health is a strong indicator of generalized health pointing toward longevity and optimal performance of all the body's metabolic systems. Colon health is enhanced by a number of factors such as increasing the quantity of fruits and vegetables in the diet, higher fiber consumption, adequate hydration, colon cleansing, and probiotic supplementation. It has often been said, and it should be regarded as truth, that good health begins in the colon. As much as the topic of bowel hygiene might be squeamish, it is very important if the goal is good nutrition, optimal health, and longevity.

The rich density of "friendly" bacteria in the gut can be affected by numerous processes. There can be no denying that the *Standard American Diet* has proven as damaging to our lower digestive tract as it is to the integrity of other body systems. Among the many benefits of healthy gut microbiome is preventing constipation, which creates a myriad of toxic effects. Some *100 trillion* friendly bacteria inhabit the average human gut where they are responsible for breaking down dense proteins, increasing levels of *polyamines (PA's)* in the gut, as well as helping to displace *unfriendly* bacteria and parasites within the digestive tract. Intestinal PA's are important chemicals in mammals which help to prevent chronic low-grade inflammation, a key marker of aging and overall immune health. Low levels of polyamines are closely "associated with intestinal barrier dysfunction" (constipation) One study concluded that treatment of laboratory mice with probiotic bacteria resulted in increased longevity which was associated with the "suppression of chronic low-grade inflammation in the colon induced by higher PA level," thereby concluding that simple probiotic supplementation was an easily available approach to increase lifespan. [114]

---

[114] Longevity in mice is promoted by probiotic-induced suppression of colonic senescence dependent on upregulation of gut bacterial polyamine production., Matsumoto et. al., August 2011, from PLos One / PubMed, indexed for MEDLINE

Another study, published in *Nature Communications*, compared the standard Western diet with those of African populations and concluded that "A traditional African diet is high in fibre and low in fat, with plenty of fruits, vegetables, beans and cornmeal, and very little meat", resulting in significantly lowered risk of cardiovascular disease and colon cancer due to the proliferation of a healthy gut environment. [115]

If our desire is to live longer and healthier, we cannot ignore this body of science which supports optimizing the health of the colon. Natural strategies which include colon cleansing, probiotic supplementation, *avoidance* of pharmaceutical antibiotics, increased consumption of insoluble fiber, and parasite cleansing, are vital components of a lifelong set of strategies for overall health; particularly in the colon.

---

[115] African diet may help lower the risk of colon cancer, says new study, by DN2 Team, from the Kenya Daily Nation, May 2016

# Appendix 3 – **Three Critical Blood Hormones Critical to Aging**

In this brief sketch, we look at 3 primary blood markers for their potential harm or benefit toward healthy aging. All of these are the consequence of controllable environmental and lifestyle factors. By doing the right thing, we achieve an optimal outcome. Yet, most of us will likely never pay attention to these important endocrine system markers.

**Homocysteine** – Homocysteine is a common amino acid (one of the building blocks that make up proteins) found in the blood and in *most* people is acquired from eating meat. High levels of plasma homocysteine are indicative of the advance of a cardiovascular disease. It is part of the methylation cycle and helps to create reactions that aid DNA and RNA metabolism. Elevated levels of homocysteine in the blood are commonly associated with atherosclerosis, increases in clumping of blood plasma cells, Alzheimer's disease, depression, menopause symptoms, arthritis, and heart disease. Though blood levels of homocysteine are expected to increase with age, we now know that they can be regulated, thereby reducing the risk of heart disease. Trimethylglycine (TMG), derived from sugar beets, is an effective supplement that modulates homocysteine levels by donating methyl components. Vitamins B6 and B12 are critical supplements that help to modulate homocysteinemia. Nori (a sea vegetable) is another great source of vitamin B12 along with fermented foods.

**C-Reactive Protein (CRP)** – Testing for this blood protein measures general levels of inflammation in the body. High measurement of CRP within the body is closely associated with the risk of cardiovascular incident (heart attack), stroke, high cholesterol levels, and inflammation in the cells which line the arteries. Chronic low-grade inflammation is a consistent marker of a spectrum of disorders which contribute to accelerated aging processes. Testing for plasma levels of CRP is considered to be a more effective diagnostic tool than mere cholesterol testing as predictive of cardiovascular disease risk. Other conditions associated with inflammation include allergies, asthma, eczema, autoimmune disease, diabetes, Alzheimer's and arthritis.    A diet abundant in fresh vegetables and fruits, along with supplements such as Vitamin E and DHEA, are ideal ways to reduce levels of CRP in the blood.

**Endorphins** – These are a group of *endogenous peptides* (chemicals made within the body) found in the brain that bind to opiate receptors and produces pain-relief effects similar to that of opiates.  Specifically considered a *neuropeptide*, endorphins are part of the neuronal signaling molecules that communicate between neurons.  There are multiple ways to increase health-enhancing levels of endorphins, including exercise, eating chocolate and chili peppers, making love, massage therapy, meditation, and laughter.

# Appendix 4 – **Water is Life, Dehydration is Death**

Since the dawn of life on this planet, water has always had a direct relationship to Life. We must maintain a proper ratio of brain hydration to enjoy optimal mental function. It is also true that overheating water challenges its oxygen-carrying capacity. And how many of us are aware that eating cooked food requires higher levels of water consumption? The science on H2O is much deeper than most of us might imagine.

- "Water represents a critical nutrient whose absence will be lethal within days. Water's importance for the prevention of nutrition-related noncommunicable diseases has emerged more recently because of the shift toward large proportions of fluids coming from caloric beverages... Water comprises from 75% body weight in infants to 55% in elderly and is essential for cellular homeostasis and life." – *Water, Hydration and Health*, by authors Popkin, D'Anci and Rosenberg

- "Further, dehydration prevents accumulations from being washed out of the cells and tissues. These accumulations, such as cholesterol, lactic-acid wastes, pyruvic crystals, or calcium, muck up the cell membranes, clog the efficient pathways of arteries and inhibit the smooth motion of the joint capsules; and thus contribute to such chronic degenerative diseases as arteriosclerosis, arthritis, gout, kidney stones and gallstones, to name a few. ¶Water is the substance that takes the toxins and carbon dioxide out and carries vital nutrients in. That is why it can and should be considered an anti-aging remedy!" – *Water – For Life and Anti-Aging*, by Donna Gates, BodyEcology.com

- "As people age the majority of them tend to dehydrate. The average adult's body is around 75% water but people in old age or who have a chronic illness can dip as low as 65% for men and 52% for women. At the brink of death, this can drop another 10%. Dehydration and its correlation with dead things are synonymous throughout nature. Think of plants and leaves that are dead. They dry up and become brittle and fragile. Most people literally shrink and dry up as they age past a certain point (wrinkles, loss of height and muscle mass) due to severe chronic dehydration from not getting the benefits of drinking water daily... ¶ The brain is 85% water. When dehydration is taking place and this percentage drops even just a small amount, the brain begins to have trouble dealing with multiple inputs. The result is a person who becomes depressed from feeling overwhelmed and *unable to handle life*". – Govan Kilgour, *Secrets of Longevity*

- "In advanced societies, thinking that tea, coffee, alcohol, and manufactured beverages are desirable substitutes for the purely natural water needs of the daily 'stressed' body is an elementary but catastrophic mistake. It is true that these beverages contain water, but what else they contain are dehydrating agents. They get rid of the water they are dissolved in plus some more water from the reserves of the body! Today's modern lifestyle makes people dependent on all sorts of beverages that are commercially manufactured." – *Your Body's Many Cries for Water*, by F. Batmanghelidj, M.D.

- "As we get older, body water content decreases, the risk for dehydration increases, and the consequences become more serious. Dehydration has been associated with increased mortality rates among hospitalized older adults and can precipitate emergency hospitalization and increases the risk of repeated stays in a hospital. Dehydration is a frequent cause of hospitalization of older adults and one of the ten most frequent diagnoses responsible for hospitalization in the United States. Evidence suggests high dehydration rates of elderly patients within hospitals and other health care institutions. Dehydration has also been associated with various morbidities, such as impaired cognition or acute confusion, falling or constipation. The cost associated with dehydration may be very high: a study conducted in 1999 in the United States evaluated the avoidable costs of hospitalizations due to dehydration at $1.14 billion." – *Hydration and the Elderly*, from the H4H Initiative Newsletter

# Appendix 5 – **Protecting Children from Before Conception to Infancy**

Few of us might imagine the impact of the very first stages and staging of life as directly related to longevity. Yet, preconception, in utero and early infancy can all affect longevity and quality of life. One can examine these three stages in detail and realize just how many things can go wrong during each of these critical stages of life.

## Preconception

Before conception, a multiplicity of effects can occur to both women and men which can have a significant impact on the fetus and throughout the child's life. Mothers can be affected by a number of exposures to toxicants which harm the developing ova. These can include radiation exposure, hormonally active agents (endocrine disrupting chemicals), alcohol, cigarettes, PCB's, furan exposure in cooking oil, and other persistent pollutants. Similarly, many of these same exposures can damage men's sperm-producing capacity or can have damaging effects on the male's chromosomes which are then paired with female chromosomes in the conjoining of egg and sperm to form the fertilized embryo. It has long been shown that alcohol abuse can compromise sperm DNA and studies on the impact of common pharmaceutical drugs have linked them to male infertility and sperm damage.

## Abortion and miscarriage shorten the maternal lifespan

Two studies compared life expectancy between women who had given birth to others, whose pregnancies were interrupted due to abortion, miscarriage, as well as combinations of these outcomes; the studies demonstrated that multiple interruptions compounded the risk of early death. Findings among the two studies were consistent and showed that: "With controls for the number of pregnancies, year of birth, and age at last pregnancy, when compared to only giving birth, having only induced abortion(s) was associated with a 66% increased risk of dying. A reproductive history entailing only natural losses (compared to birth) was associated with a 181% increased risk of dying across the study period... ¶

Multiple abortions, compared to no experience of abortion, and after applying controls, increased the risk of mortality as follows: one abortion, 45%; two abortions, 114%; three abortions, 191%. Similarly, increased risks of death were equal to 44%, 86%, and 150% for one, two, and three natural losses respectively compared to no natural losses." The mechanisms associated with this negative outcome are associated with *posttraumatic stress syndrome* yet could also be associated with the hormonal disruption caused by interruption of pregnancy.

## Endocrine disorders and pregnancy infections

Throughout history, pregnant women were not exposed to the spectrum of food-borne and environmental stressors that exist today. Their developing fetuses were not bombarded with endocrine disrupting chemicals, electromagnetic radiation, ultrasound microwaves, along with a range of foods which are increasingly unfit for pregnant mothers. We all have heard, for good reason, that pregnant women must avoid alcohol, smoking, and exposure to volatile chemicals.

There is a spectrum of exposures that women are currently experiencing which are proving to be damaging with sometimes gross and sometimes subtle effects. *"Intercurrent disease"* in pregnancy is not regarded as a "complication of pregnancy" but relates to disease conditions that occur during pregnancy. These can include endocrine disorders such as *gestational diabetes* and thyroid disease. As you realize by now, the Standard American Diet is notoriously *diabetogenic*. Naturally-produced pregnancy hormones can increase thyroid hormone levels in the blood (*hyperthyroidism*) and this effect can be compounded by other stressors. Drugs used to treat these conditions, along with other infections, disorders, chronic diseases, and autoimmune conditions, are risky to the developing fetus, depending on the mechanism of the drugs taken.

According to the growing mass of research on the topic, avoiding pharmaceutical drugs, as well as with alcohol, smoking, and street drugs, is the best advice to be offered – not only during pregnancy but in pre-pregnancy and during lactation.

## Early childhood stress, toxicity and drug dependency

As with natural pregnancy – aside from historic dangers from infectious diseases that were largely attributed to underdeveloped hygienic facilities – under proper environmental conditions, children will grow up strong and healthy, benefiting from the evolutionary inheritance passed to their generation from 3 million years of human genetic refinement. Yet, sadly, we are witnessing the rise of a spectrum of childhood disorders and diseases that is truly a national tragedy; especially when we consider the wealth and technological capacity of this nation. Infectious diseases that have caused the bulk of childhood deaths over the centuries are now replaced by *non-communicable diseases*, immune disorders, diabetes, overweight, autism, and other mental disorders, as well as the numerous effects of a sedentary childhood preoccupied with electronic recreation. Breastfeeding is increasingly being displaced by laboratory-concocted formulas, which are known to contain allergy-producing proteins, gender-bending chemicals and worse, and this toxic mess is even being served up in baby bottles that expose infants to dangerous petrochemical endocrine disruptors; made worse when plastic baby bottles are heated in a microwave oven. Rising alarms about early childhood vaccinations can no longer be ignored as the U.S. vaccine schedule is many times more intense than that of other developed nations; many families have chosen to forego vaccine injections completely. As well, childhood nutrition, served in the home and at school, is over processed, lacking essential nutrient groups, and overloaded with sugar, fat and allergy-provoking dairy products. Cancer among children, rare in previous centuries, is now an increasing risk worldwide.

## Which way forward?

Where do we go from where we are? We would like to believe that ours is a rational, resourceful and caring generation. Yet, the way this nation treats its childbearing-age youth, pregnant mothers and young children does not reflect the highest qualities of a civilized society. It's not as if the wisdom to do better doesn't exist; to the contrary, high-quality science has supported efforts by genuinely caring individuals and organizations at every level of society who just are not getting the support they need from government and health agencies. We don't seem to understand just why it is so important to protect our progeny as we project them into the future.

It is my great hope and intention that what you have just read will become a major influence in your thoughts, values, and actions within your own family and for the larger society.

# Appendix 6 – **Notes on Devolution**

## DNA Methylation and Chromosomal Damage

Since I first advanced this concept of *Evolution Verses Devolution*, I have been carrying it in my conscious mind as I move through and examine the world around me. I am coming more and more to see this as a breakthrough hypothesis in examining various fields of microbiology, genetics, environmental science as well as both social and political affairs.

To re-establish my central premise here, because of a spectrum of environmental stresses, happening throughout life, during pregnancy as well before conception, our generation is witnessing the conjoining of environmental factors that are changing the very nature of our species. Homo sapiens is splitting into two evolutionary lines.

So many people are being injured by these toxic stressors that they are now giving birth to children (or *not*, in the case of reproductive failure) that are genetically less viable than the parent generation. As well, this is happening on such scale that the patterns of genetic downgrading are being pushed into the future as a branch of the human species breaking off from the *idealized* evolutionary inheritance of modern man.

Evolution is supposed to produce the best of the best inherited from previous generations. As Mike Judge advanced in his 2006 farcical comedy, *Idiocracy*, we may not be too far from a future where a significant portion of the population, perhaps even the majority, has lost significant function of key parts of its brain and may not even be capable of higher reasoning within the most advanced parts of the brain such as the cerebral cortex, hippocampus and the most recent part of the human brain to evolve, the *pre-frontal cortex*.

What I am putting forward herein is that this corruption is happening even before conception. A damaged parental-gene donor, whose chromosomes have been corrupted, along with the procedural functioning that regulates gene expression (called methylation), can thus transmit chromosomal insufficiency into the egg, sperm cell and fertilized zygote which are then passed on into the next generation at fertilization.

Both male and female donate to the embryo 23 pairs of chromosomes each as half of the needed 46 chromosome pairs which comprise a whole person. The process by which each of the gender's bodies split their own 46 chromosome pairs into half is called *meiosis*. If, going into meiosis, the material has been damaged or the process for the splitting has become errant, then the resultant sperm, in the case of the male, or egg, in the case of the female, can very likely be altered, damaged or otherwise maladapted on the very DNA level.

The process by which DNA coding is expressed in the broad spectrum of life processes is regulated by *methylation*; which is present in all life forms. Methylation is instigated by the influence of the methyl molecule ($CH_3$ – one carbon atom bound to three hydrogen atoms; an alkyl radical derived from methane). Methylation is what gives "life" to DNA, which without this process, is inert genetic *potential*. Methylation is ultimately controlled by other molecular biological processes as a function of *epigenetics*, which modern genetics researchers consider to be near the cutting edge of microbiology, biogenetics and the environmental regulation of gene expression. The frontier of this research is also bridging epigenetics and *quantum physics*, a topic we have explored at length elsewhere in this book.

I will have much more to study before I can completely teach on this subject of methylation and DNA. Here are a few excerpts from the materials I have assembled as I continue to examine the topic in depth.

- **DNA methylation** – "is an epigenetic mechanism used by cells to control gene expression. A number of mechanisms exist to control gene expression in eukaryotes, but DNA methylation is a commonly used epigenetic signaling tool that can fix genes in the "off" position. ¶ Over recent decades, scientists have made various discoveries about DNA methylation and how vital it is to a number of cellular processes such as embryonic development, X-chromosome inactivation, genomic imprinting, gene suppression, carcinogenesis, and chromosome stability. Researchers have linked abnormal DNA methylation to several adverse outcomes, including human diseases." [116]

- **DNA methylation** – "is an epigenetic mechanism that occurs by the addition of a methyl (CH3) group to DNA, thereby often modifying the function of the genes. The most widely characterized DNA methylation process is the covalent addition of the methyl group at the 5-carbon of the cytosine ring resulting in 5-methylcytosine (5-mC), also informally known as the "fifth base" of DNA. These methyl groups project into the major groove of DNA and inhibit transcription." [117]

- **The Role of Methylation in Gene Expression** – "In recent decades, researchers have learned a great deal about DNA methylation, including how it occurs and where it occurs, and they have also discovered that methylation is an important component in numerous cellular processes, including embryonic development, genomic imprinting, X-chromosome inactivation, and preservation of chromosome stability. Given the many processes in which methylation plays a part, it is perhaps not surprising that researchers have also linked errors in methylation to a variety of devastating consequences, including several human diseases." [118]

- **The New Physics: Planting Both Feet Firmly on Thin Air** – Author Bruce Lipton, Ph.D. writes: "Reviewing this ground-breaking study for Nature, biophysicist F. Weinhold concluded: 'When will chemistry textbooks begin to serve as aids, rather than barriers, to this enriched quantum-mechanic perspective on how molecular turnstiles work?' He further emphasized: 'What are the forces that control the twisting and folding of molecules into complex shapes? Don't look for the answers in your organic chemistry textbook.' Yet organic chemistry provides the mechanistic foundation for biomedicine; and as Weinhold notes, that branch of science is so far out of date that its textbooks have yet to recognize quantum

---

[116] What is DNA Methylation?, By Sally Robertson, BSc, News Medical Life Sciences & Medicine, news-medical.net

[117] DNA Methylation, from What is Epigenetics? / author unattributed, WhatIsEpigenetics.com

[118] The Role of Methylation in Gene Expression, By: Theresa Phillips, Ph.D., Nature Education / Citation: Phillips, T. (2008)

mechanics. Conventional medical researchers have no understanding of the molecular mechanisms that truly provide for life." [119]

- **Meiosis** – "Chromosome abnormalities usually happen as a result of an error in cell division. Meiosis is the name used to describe the cell division that the egg and sperm undergo when they are developing. Normally, meiosis causes a halving of chromosome material, so that each parent gives 23 chromosomes to a pregnancy. ¶ The result is an egg or sperm with only 23 chromosomes. When fertilization occurs, the normal 46 total number of chromosomes results in the fetus. If meiosis does not occur properly, an egg or sperm could end up with too many chromosomes, or not enough chromosomes. Upon fertilization, the baby could then receive an extra chromosome (called a trisomy) or have a missing chromosome (called a monosomy)." [120]

- **Impact of DNA Damage on the Frequency of Sperm Chromosomal Aneuploidy in Normal and Subfertile Men** – "Sperm nuclear defects might be the reason for a worldwide increasing trend of male infertility in terms of average low sperm counts and sperm quality in developed countries. Sperm cells carry a demonstrable background level of aneuploidy [when a cell has an abnormal number of chromosomes other than 46 in human cells] and chromosome breakage; however, a number of risk factors might lead to increase this baseline. ¶ The causes of sperm DNA damage, much like those of male infertility, have many factors and may be attributed to interior extra testicular factors (i.e. drugs, chemotherapy, radiation therapy, cigarette smoking, environmental toxins, genital tract inflammation, testicular hyperthermia, varicocele, hormonal factors and so on). Sperm DNA damage is clearly associated with male infertility (and abnormal spermatogenesis), but a small percentage

---

[119] The Biology of Belief: Unleashing the power of consciousness, matter & miracles, by Bruce H. Lipton, Ph.D., Pgs 110-111
[120] How Chromosome Abnormalities Happen: Meiosis, Mitosis, Maternal Age, Environment, from the Health Encyclopedia, University of Rochester Medical Center

of spermatozoa from fertile men also possesses detectable levels of DNA damage." [121]

As you can certainly tell by now, the science that can be brought to bear to support my unique and radical hypothesis that humanity is in danger of splitting into two groups, the genetic *haves,* and *have-nots*, is supported by multiple processes by which our chromosomes are being challenged. The identifying labels I am proposing for these divergent groups are the *Evolutionaries* and the less fortunate *Devolutionaries*.

What must be noted is that the processes which are causative of this proposed split are epigenetic and thus ultimately suited for moderation by our awareness of, and action toward optimizing environmental conditions. Yet these proposed controls require our discipline and retraction from a spectrum of culturally accepted behaviors within so-called "modern society."

Whether the majority will opt to exclude corrupting influences in order to secure a distant outcome is yet to be determined. By coincidence, this is exactly the primary function of the pre-frontal cortex, that most advanced part of the brain responsible for calculating the value of delayed gratification, that is currently under greatest assault from the spectrum of interruptions. As stated before, other areas of the brain, including the hippocampus, cerebral cortex, and various glandular axes are also subject to evolutionary compromise.

---

[121] Impact of DNA Damage on the Frequency of Sperm Chromosomal Aneuploidy in Normal and Subfertile Men, Iran Biomedical Journal. 2011 Oct; 15(4): 122–129.

# Appendix 7 – **Eating for Longevity**

## Superfoods Facilitate High-Quality Life Extension

1. Our bodies have a need for 8 basic classes of nutrition; they are hydration, vitamins, minerals, protein (source of amino acids), essential fatty acids, fiber, carbohydrates, and enzymes.

2. Not only do we need these critical nutrients, but we must also optimize the way that we access them. Many modern food preparation methods and technologies are destructive to the essential nature of these nutrients. As well, mass production of food introduces many unnatural elements into the food chain which are potentially harmful.

3. The structural design of the human body is optimized for digesting fruits, vegetables, nuts, whole grains, and seeds – all representing a plant-based diet.

4. Functional Medicine is the medical practice of using nutrition to prevent disease by eradicating the foundation of pathogenesis (injury creation). The term was coined by Jeffrey Bland, Ph.D., co-founder of the Institute for Functional Medicine.

5. Clinical Nutrition is the medical practice of using nutrition, in the form of juices, plant-based foods, and healing herbs, as the primary means of triggering the body's endogenous (internal) healing capabilities to overcome disease and disorder.

6. Superfoods are a class of foods known to have the densest concentration of the 8 basic classes of nutrients. They can be broadly classified as greens, nuts & seeds, sea vegetables, tropical fruits, and hydrating foods.

7. David Wolfe's book **SUPERFOODS: The Food and Medicine of the Future**, lists the top 10 superfoods as:

   a. Goji berries

   b. Cacao (raw chocolate)

   c. Maca (the Andes aphrodisiac)

   d. Bee products, including honey, bee pollen, royal jelly, and propolis

   e. Spirulina (best source of protein of any food)

   f. AFA Blue-Green Algae (super blue-green algae), grown in Klamath Lake, Oregon

   g. Marine Phytoplankton – the root of all sea life and source of omega 3 in seafood

   h. Aloe Vera

   i. Hempseed and hempseed oil

   j. Coconuts – coconut water, oil, butter, jelly, dried and shredded

8. Other top superfoods include:

   a. Kale – the superfood of greens, which are an essential superfood (they contain high amounts of magnesium, a deficiency of which is associated with a long list of diseases and disorders. Spinach is the stuff that made Popeye the superhero that he became; it can do the same for all of us.

   b. Walnuts – the superfood of nuts, as well as almonds and other and seed nut butters

   c. Seeds: sunflower, sesame (tahini is sesame seed butter), pumpkin, flax & chia, beans, and lentils

   d. Apple cider vinegar

   e. Miso (organic, fermented soy paste)

   f. Cultured vegetables (raw sauerkraut and kimchi)

   g. Vegetables including carrots, cabbage, peppers, tomatoes, beets and sprouts

    h. Fruits including apples, avocados, citrus fruits, red grapes, soursop, bananas, blueberries, pomegranates, cranberries, cherries, prunes, and papaya

    i. Great immune boosting vegetables include broccoli, cauliflower, onions

    j. Powerful culinary herbs include turmeric, cinnamon, curry, cayenne pepper, ginger, and garlic

9. Great oils include hemp seed oil, flax oil, avocado oil, sunflower oil, safflower oil, olive oil, walnut oil, sesame seed oil. BAD OILS include hydrogenated oils, canola (GMO), vegetable oil, corn oil (GMO) and *blended* oils.

10. Foods that protect from toxic heavy metals – Amino acids (commonly obtained from meat and eggs) can be obtained from eating seeds and nuts; cilantro, activated charcoal, Brazil nuts, onions & garlic, and chlorella

11. Top brain foods, herbs, and supplements that prevent the degeneration of memory, and combat dementia and Alzheimer's disease include ginkgo biloba, Gotu kola, green juicing, sea vegetables, melons (watermelon, cantaloupe, jackfruit), papaya, blueberries, walnuts, kidney beans, wheatgrass, ginger, and cinnamon.

# BIBLIOGRAPHY – Critical Reading on Longevity and Natural Health

Here I share a list of must-read books which allow us insight into the manner by which Nature and science have allowed us to master longevity and avoid disease. These include studies by some of the world's foremost natural health researchers, healers, microbiologists, pioneers on the frontier of scientific discovery and those involved in clinical medicine at all levels. I include five of my own books in this list as well.

- Living Super In Paradise: Creating Space for Perfect Health
- Living Superfood Recipes: Medicine Has Never Tasted Like This Before – Keidi Awadu
- Living Superfood Recipes Vol 2: Food is Nature's Most Perfect Medicine – Keidi Awadu
- Living Superfood Research: Don't Get Sick, Stay Off Drugs and Live a Long Time – Keidi Awadu
- Soul Food: Do We Really Know What's in It? – Keidi Awadu
- Get the Weight Off: 30 Days to a New You – Keidi Awadu
- Epidemic: The Rise of New Childhood Diseases in the U.S. (A Man-Made Disaster) – Keidi Awadu
- Gary Null's Mind Power: Rejuvenate Your Brain and Memory Naturally
- Reverse the Aging Process Naturally – Dr. Gary Null, PhD
- Power Foods for the Brain – Neal D. Barnard
- Rainbow Green Live-Food Cuisine – Dr. Gabriel Cousens
- Conscious Eating – Dr. Gabriel Cousens
- Superfoods: The Food and Medicine of the Future – David Wolfe

- The Gerson Therapy: The Proven Nutritional Program for Cancer and Other Illnesses – Charlotte Gerson and Morton Walker

- The Longevity Bible – Gary Small, M.D.

- Healthy Aging – Dr. Andrew Weil, M.D.

- Stopping the Clock: Longevity for the New Millennium – Ronald Klatz and Robert Goldman

- Soak Your Nuts: Cleansing with Karyn – Karyn Calabrese

- Super Foods for Seniors – FC&A Medical Publishing

- OXYGEN: The Molecule that Made the World – Nick Lane

- The Biology of Belief – Bruce H. Lipton, Ph.D.

- Life Extension Magazine – www.LifeExtension.com

## INDEX